The Female Pelvis
Anatomy and Exercises

The Female Pelvis

Anatomy & Exercises

BLANDINE CALAIS-GERMAIN

EASTLAND PRESS ❖ SEATTLE

Originally published in French as *Le périnée féminin* by Éditions DésIris.

P.O. Box 99749, Seattle, WA 98139 USA

ISBN-10: 0-939616-38-6
ISBN-13: 978-0-939616-38-1
Library of Congress Control Number: 2002102916
Printed in the United States of America

4 6 8 10 9 7 5 3

English language edition translated by Blandine Calais-Germain, edited by Allan Kaplan

Book design by Gary Niemeier

J'oublais … Par des fleurs,
Par des saules cache,
Jalousement gardé,
Un puits, soif et fraîcheur,
Qui s'exalte à la pluie,
Draine leas forces vives,
De l'ume à l'autre rive
Et fait jaillir la vie …

I had forgotten… A well
hidden amongst flowers
and willows,
jealously guarded.
A well of freshness and thirst
that exults and swells with rain,
pulling toward itself
from each bank
vital forces which
burst into life…

—Bernard Haillant
extract from the song *Ma province*

THIS BOOK provides three types of information:

- *Explanation* (pp. 12-93) of the functional anatomy of the pelvic region, and how it responds to childbirth.
- *Exercises* (pp. 94-138) for self-discovery, flexibility, strengthening, and coordination of the pelvic region.
- *Guidelines* (pp. 139-146) which focus on the pelvis during particular phases of a woman's life cycle.

Table of Contents

Foreword

THIS BOOK IS written for women during all phases of their lives, with a special emphasis on pregnancy and childbirth, when the perineum is of particular concern. In these pages you will discover a part of your body that is often ignored or misunderstood, and for that reason, often mistreated.

During childbirth the female perineum is subjected to extreme stretching and pressure. It is an experience which, even if short, can have important effects and lasting consequences. With just a little knowledge and attention, however, this region of the body can be well cared for. Before, during, and after childbirth there are certain things to do and certain things to avoid.

Later, particularly during menopause, important changes can once again modify the shape and function of the pelvic region. Yet it is possible to prepare oneself for, and thereby have a positive experience from, these changes.

The language used in this book was chosen to make the subject accessible to a wide audience. While medically accurate, I have chosen words and expressions that are closer to everyday use.

This book is addressed to physicians, physical therapists, midwives, and all associated health professionals. It is intended to be more than just another textbook. Rather, it is designed to serve as a tool to present and share information which the practitioner does not always have time to explain. Practitioners may well find this practical pedagogical approach—the result of long experience teaching physical movement—to be helpful in their work with women.

This book should be viewed in the context of up-to-date research in urology, gynecology, and proctology. It recommends a body-awareness approach that is based on a good knowledge of anatomy which is accessible to a general audience.

Work on the perineal region is integrated into work on the body as a whole, resulting in a type of attention to the care of the body which will enhance the health and function of the perineum itself.

The limitations of this book must also be clearly understood, particularly with regard to the exercises. All of the recommended exercises are based on the assumption that the woman is in good health (non-pathological context). With certain clearly marked exceptions, most of the exercises are entirely without risk. However, should a woman be particularly unfamiliar with her body, or suffer from an ailment or injury (a degree of pathology), the exercises may be impossible to perform, or may not bring about the desired results. These situations are beyond the scope of this book, and are part of the domain of medicine or therapy.

This book requires only a few hours to read straight through. However, provided that the woman has no preexisting medical problems, if the exercises are practiced for about 15 minutes each day over a period of two or three months, the results will be inestimable.

Preface

A few months ago I examined a patient who told me that after her last delivery she felt she had lost her femininity. Why? Her perineum had been torn and she suffered from urinary incontinence. She was right. Two further operations proved useless. They had even made matters worse because scarring was causing pain during sexual relations.

As a consulting gynecologist I am convinced that many patients suffer problems because they are poorly prepared for delivery, and fail to prepare the perineum during pregnancy.

Physicians, gynecologists, midwives, teachers, health educators and others engaged in health and welfare programs should, I believe, attach more importance to the perineum. It is not enough to think that a "good episiotomy" and some stitching will protect the internal pelvic structures. We all need to have a better understanding of the muscles, ligaments, and bones associated with the perineum, and of their functions.

As caregivers, we should further our efforts to help women acquire a real understanding of the perineum. Only in this way will we be able to prevent the endless complications that result from tears and lesions.

Blandine Calais-Germain has a deep knowledge of anatomy, functional and morphological. Her understanding of anatomy and movement has led to a career of teaching at schools and universities. Now, in this delightful book, she has given us a precise and serious study of the pelvis and the female perineum.

Calais-Germain's highly original approach allows women to learn about the perineum gradually, through engagement of the senses as much as the intellect. I believe that the study of this book will be both pleasurable and educational, and will provide women with a better understanding of an area of their bodies about which they are too often ignorant.

—*Dr. Joan Melendez Rusinol*
Obstetrician-Gynecologist
Department Chair, Santa Caterina Hospital
Gerona, Spain

CHAPTER ONE

The Bony Structures of the Perineum

At the lowest part of the trunk, the perineum is attached to a bony frame—the pelvis—that partially ensures its stability. To be more precise, the lower part is known as the small pelvis.

This relatively solid, fixed structure almost totally surrounds the organs and muscles of the perineum, and its solidity contrasts sharply with the great mobility of its contents. At the same time, the bones of the pelvis are able to move slightly, both against themselves and in relation to their neighbors. During this movement, the pelvis undergoes small changes in shape.

These factors—the shape of the pelvis and its slight adaptability—are important in understanding the behavior and functioning of the perineum, particularly as it relates to childbirth. In the following pages, the relationship between the shape of the pelvis and childbirth will frequently be shown and discussed.

The pelvis

This is the bony support of the perineum.

It is made up of four bones, which are arranged like a bony ring. (The pelvis is also known as the pelvic belt.)

This ring has a very sculptured appearance.

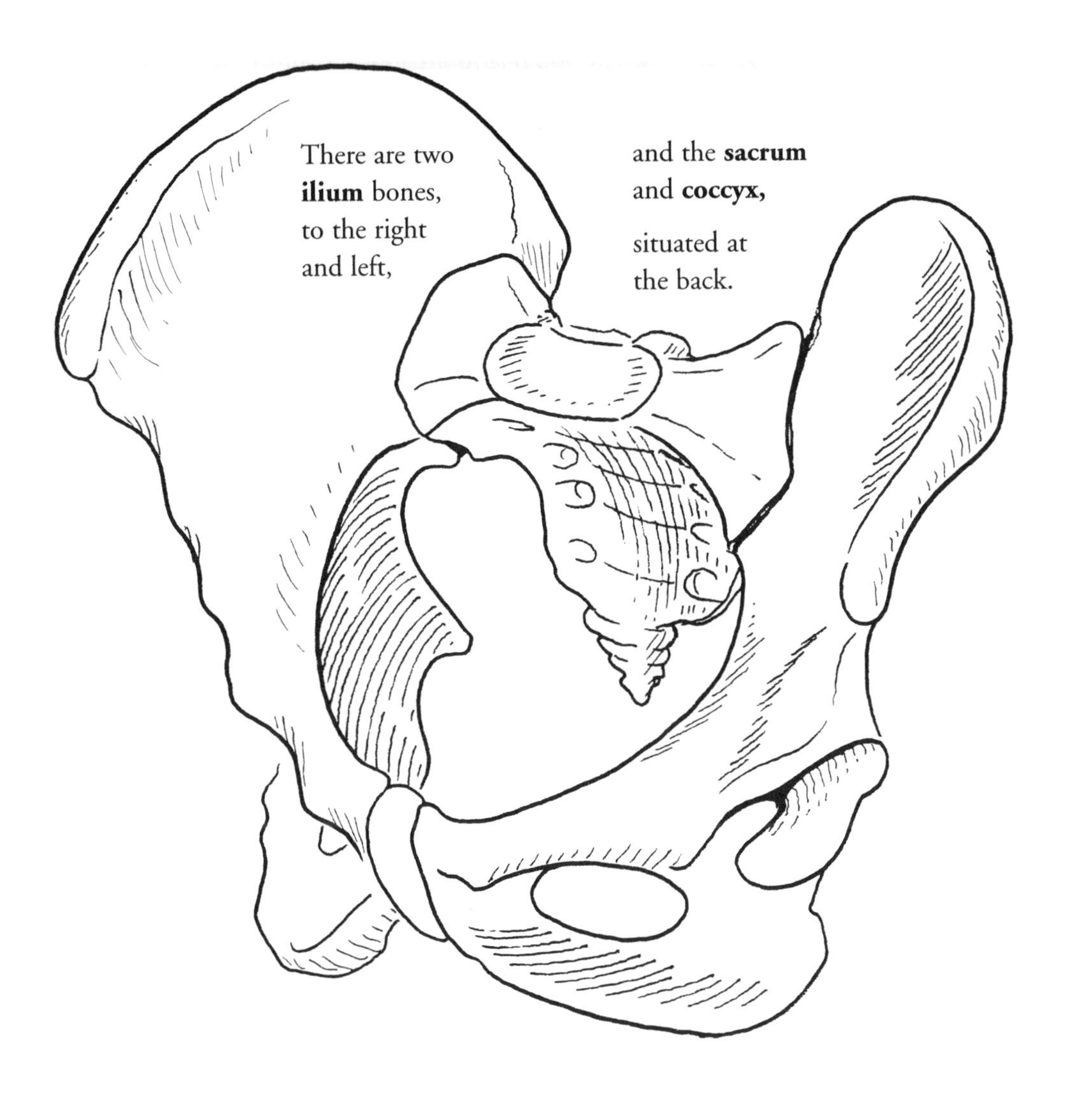

The pelvis has an internal surface—the **endopelvic** surface—that contains the pelvic organs, with the perineum at its base. An external surface—the **exopelvic** surface—corresponds to the hip joint. It is the endopelvic surface and above that is the subject of this book.

Certain parts of the pelvis can be located, allowing the reader to form a mental image of her own pelvis.

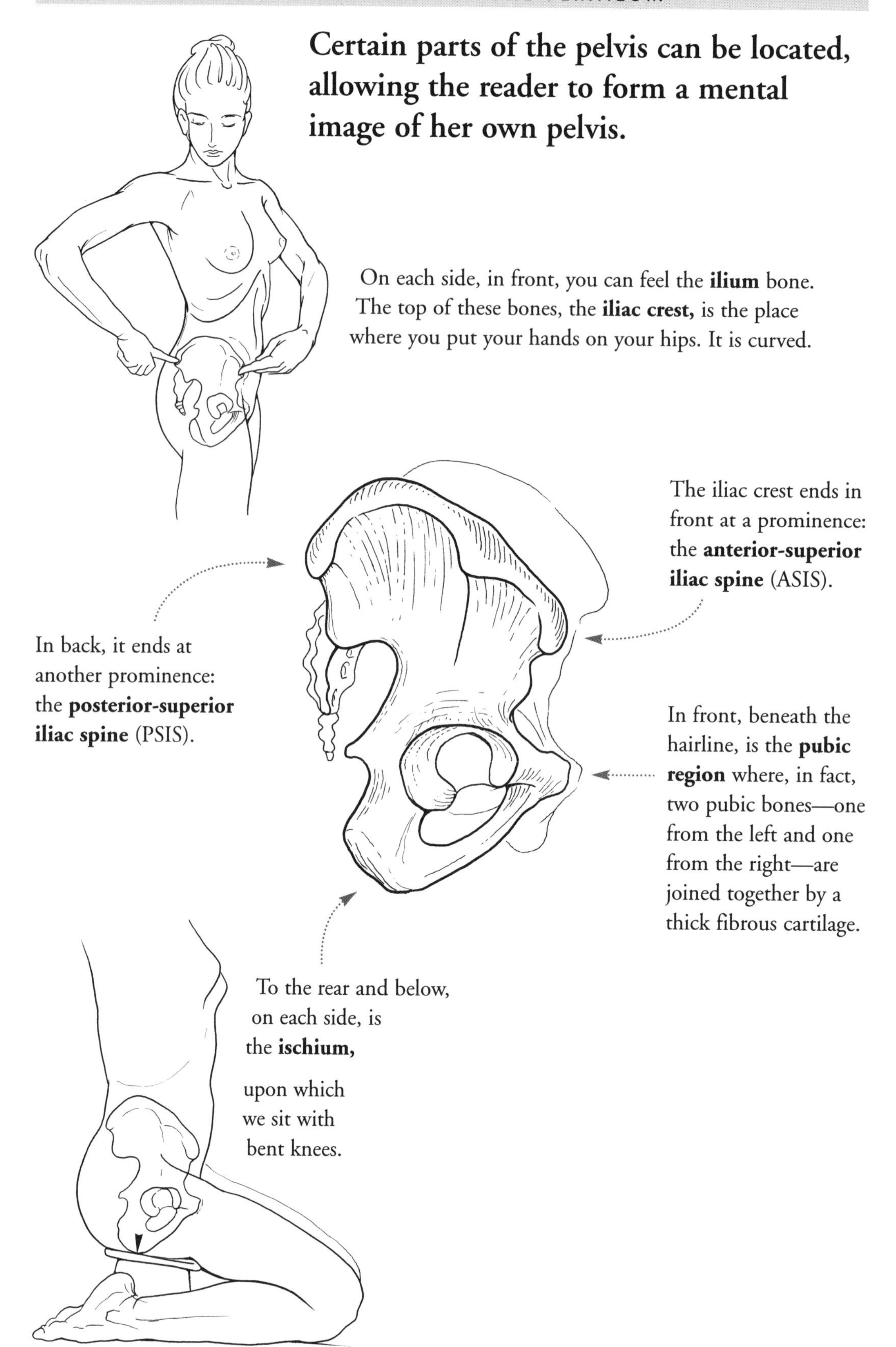

On each side, in front, you can feel the **ilium** bone. The top of these bones, the **iliac crest,** is the place where you put your hands on your hips. It is curved.

The iliac crest ends in front at a prominence: the **anterior-superior iliac spine** (ASIS).

In back, it ends at another prominence: the **posterior-superior iliac spine** (PSIS).

In front, beneath the hairline, is the **pubic region** where, in fact, two pubic bones—one from the left and one from the right—are joined together by a thick fibrous cartilage.

To the rear and below, on each side, is the **ischium,**

upon which we sit with bent knees.

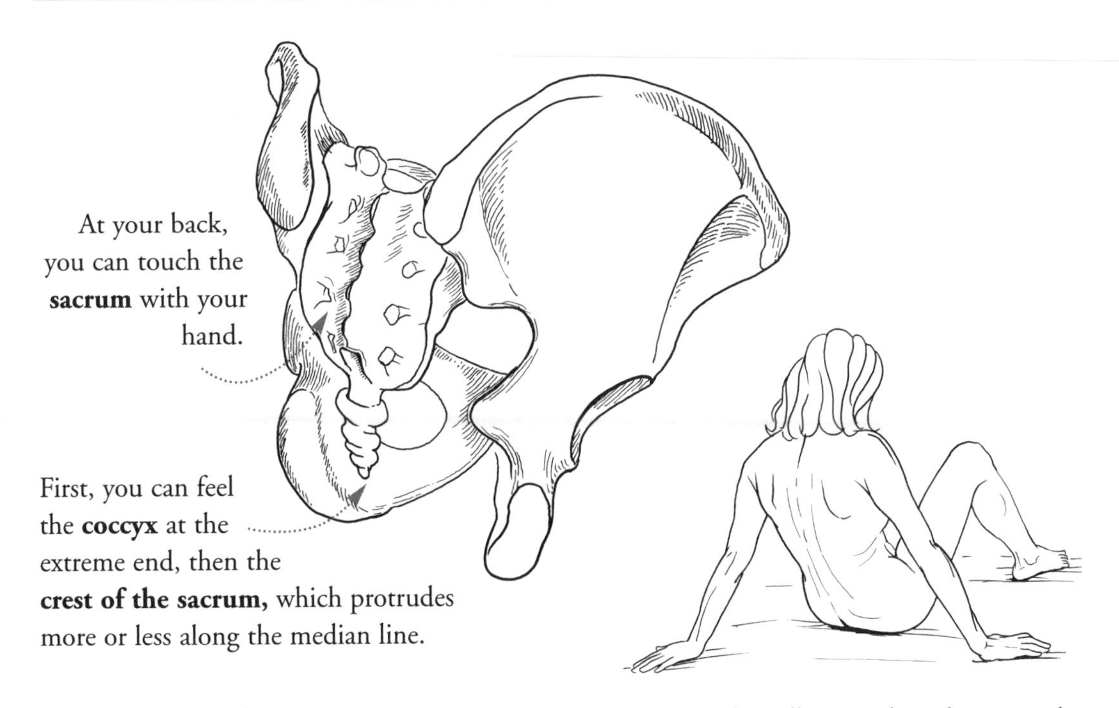

At your back, you can touch the **sacrum** with your hand.

First, you can feel the **coccyx** at the extreme end, then the **crest of the sacrum,** which protrudes more or less along the median line.

It is easier to feel the sacrum by rolling on the pelvis toward the back, using your hands as supports in order to roll gently.

Putting both hands on the iliac crests and feeling the contact made by the two ischial tuberosities on the seat below, you can get a sense of the height of your own pelvis. Form a mental image of its funnel-like shape from top to bottom.

Putting one hand on the sacrum and the other on the pubis, you can get a sense for the distance between the front and back of the pelvis.

Making the pelvis move in many different directions will give you a sense of its dimensions. This will allow you to visualize it as a bony mass that moves together as one piece.

These reference points will give you an idea of the exterior dimensions of the pelvis, and will also begin to give you an idea of its interior dimensions. Certain other reference points will be presented in the following pages.

The articulations of the pelvic bones

At the back, the sacrum articulates with each ilium bone at the **sacroiliac joint.**

On the exterior surface of the sacrum can be found a hollow surface in the shape of an upside-down "L," which is the auricle of the sacrum.

There is a corresponding articular surface on the ilium that is also L-shaped, upside down, and convex.

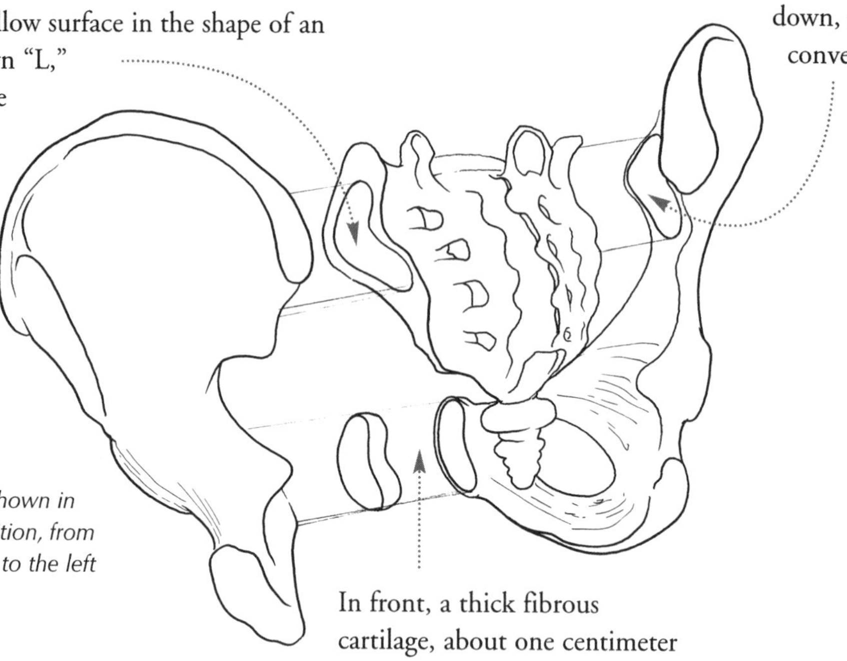

pelvis is shown in upright position, from behind and to the left

In front, a thick fibrous cartilage, about one centimeter thick,[1] joins the two pubic bones. This forms a joint called the **pubic symphysis.**

Under normal circumstances, these joints have very limited mobility, considering the shape of the surfaces involved and the presence of many ligaments, whose description is beyond the scope of this book.[2]

However, the ligaments do permit slight movement between the pelvic bones (see pp. 28-29).

During pregnancy (and also somewhat during menstruation) a flow of hormones facilitates greater movement and stretching between the two bones. This allows an increase in the pelvic diameter.

During delivery this movement becomes even greater, facilitating the delivery of the baby. This can actually be observed during the final phase of delivery by palpating the pubis with one finger.

You can prepare for the intense mobilization of the pelvis that occurs at childbirth by doing exercises (see pp. 96-101). *Note:* This preparation will not be accomplished simply by rolling the pelvis, but by performing exercises that induce actual movement between the pelvic bones.

---

1. There are about 2.5 centimeters to an inch.
2. These are described in Blandine Calais-Germain, *Anatomy of Movement* (Seattle: Eastland Press, 1993) 47, 53.

The openings

On the inside of the pelvis are a number of clearly limited zones called inlets or outlets.

These zones can be found in every female pelvis and vary in size and shape based on the proportions of the pelvic bones.

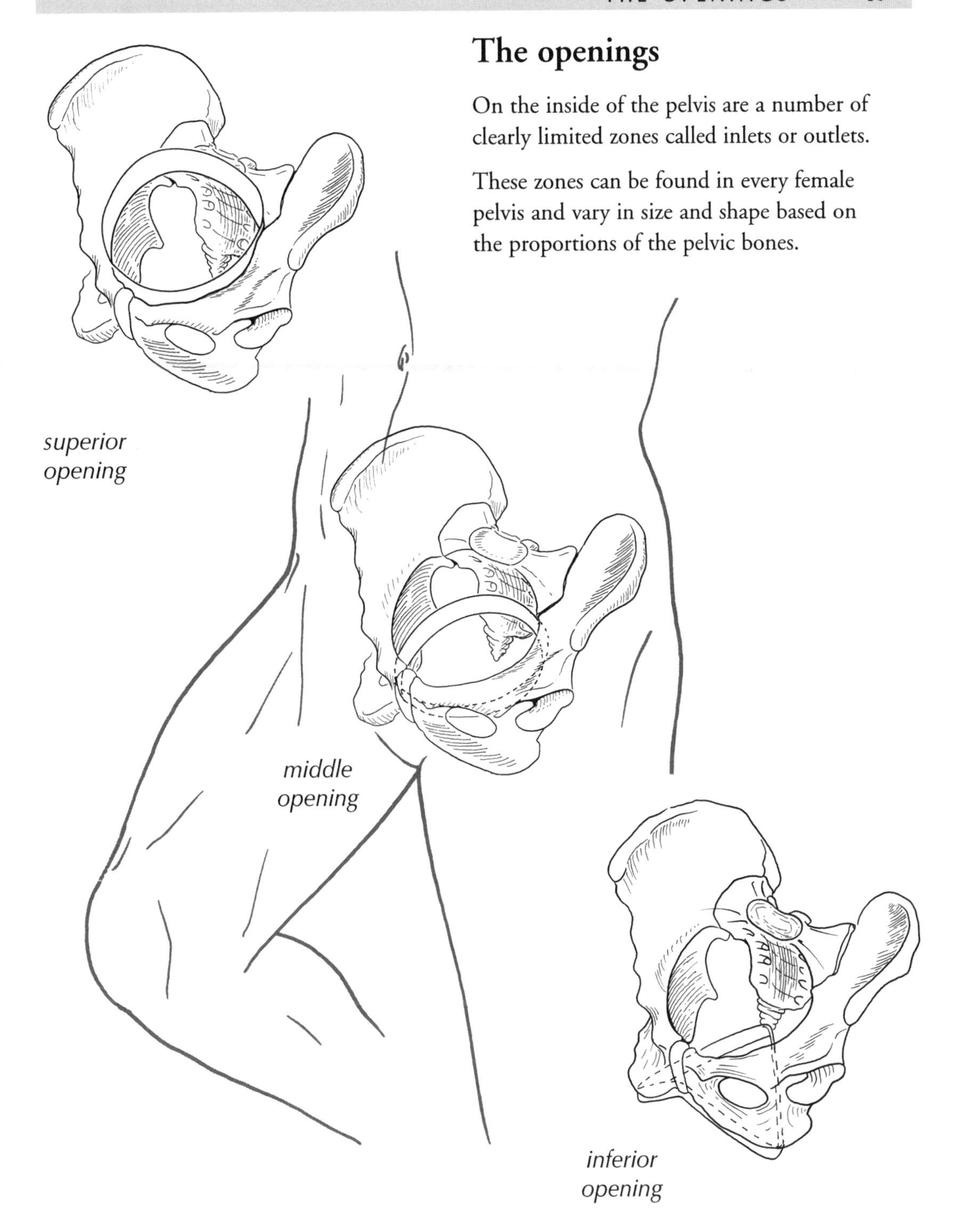

It is important to find these openings so that you can visualize:

- the points of attachment of the deep and superficial muscles of the perineum
- the shape and quality of the pelvic organs.

Moreover, the size and orientation of the openings are of extreme importance for the process of childbirth. They are described in detail in the following pages.

The superior opening

On the inner surface of the ilium bone is an oblique, curved crest that is easily recognized; this is called the **iliopectineal line.**

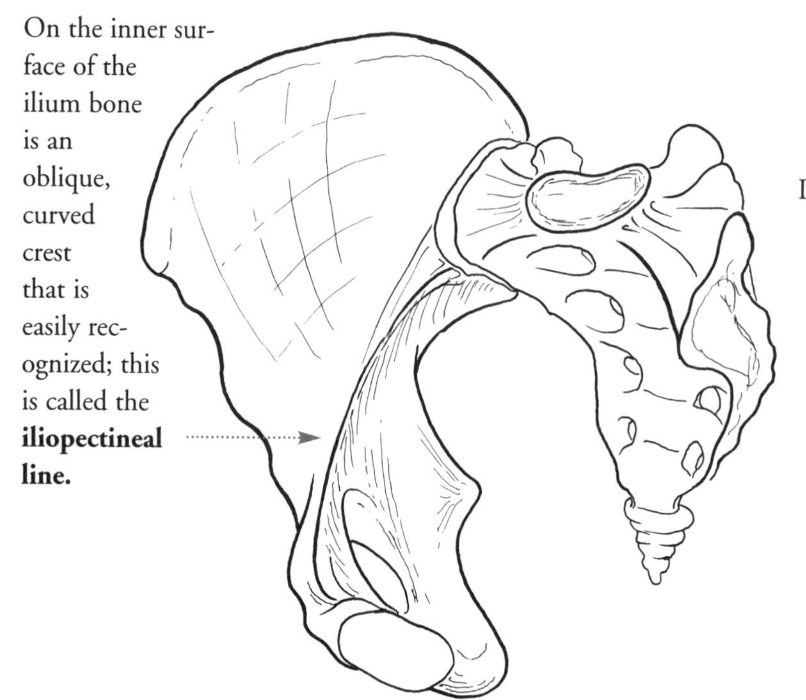

In front of the sacrum, the superior edge forms a crest called the promontory, which is extended along each side by the sacral wings.

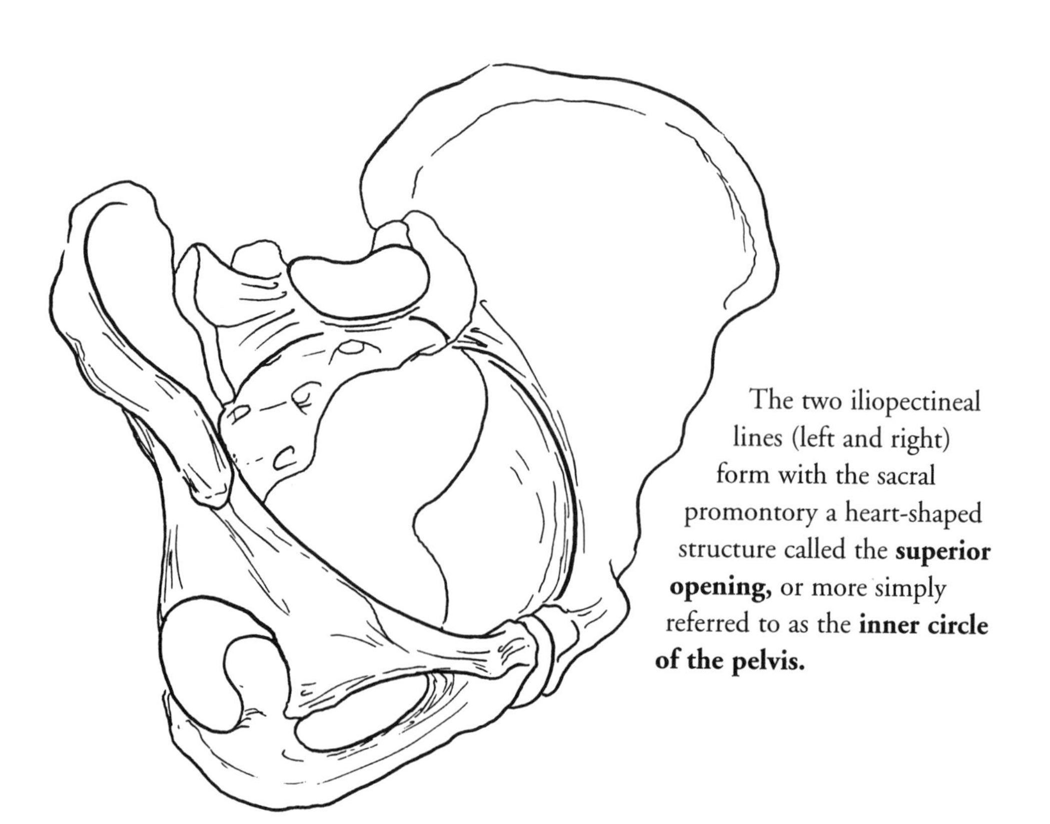

The two iliopectineal lines (left and right) form with the sacral promontory a heart-shaped structure called the **superior opening,** or more simply referred to as the **inner circle of the pelvis.**

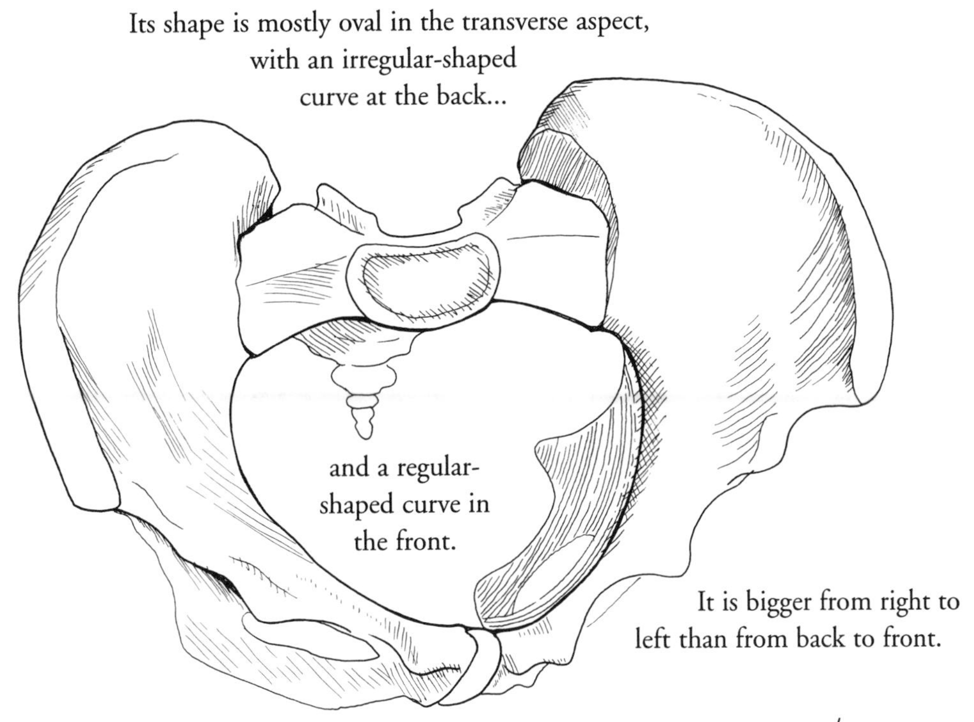

The superior opening has an oblique opening to the trunk.

When a person is in an upright position, the superior opening makes a circle higher at the back than in the front.

During delivery the superior opening is the first maternal bony passage that the fetus must pass through. At this point, it is said that the fetus "engages" with the pelvis. At the moment of engagement, the head, which until then was able to move freely, now penetrates a much narrower channel: the **lesser ("true") pelvis** (see p. 21). This leads to **rotations** (see p. 26).

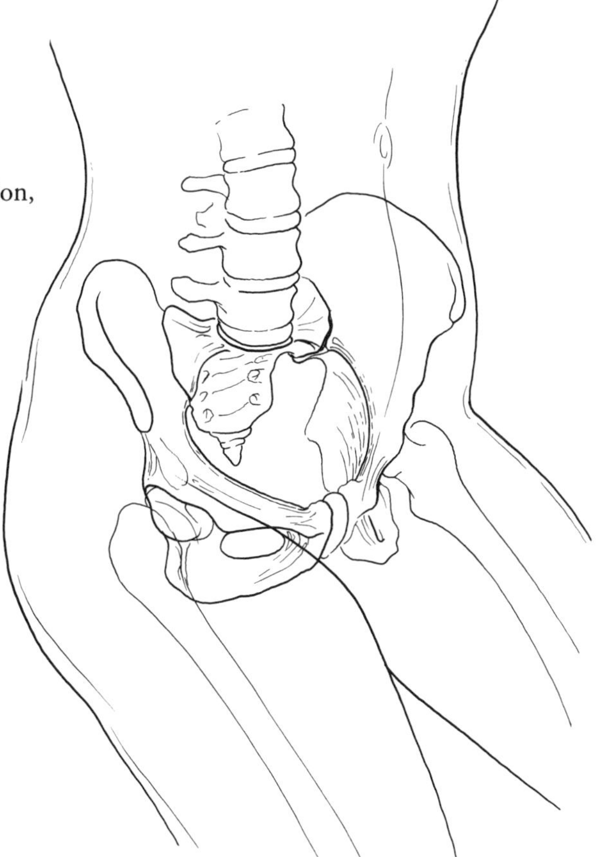

The dimensions of the superior opening are a determining factor in the delivery of the child. It is this span that is measured using a pelvimeter.

The different diameters of the superior opening are evaluated as follows:

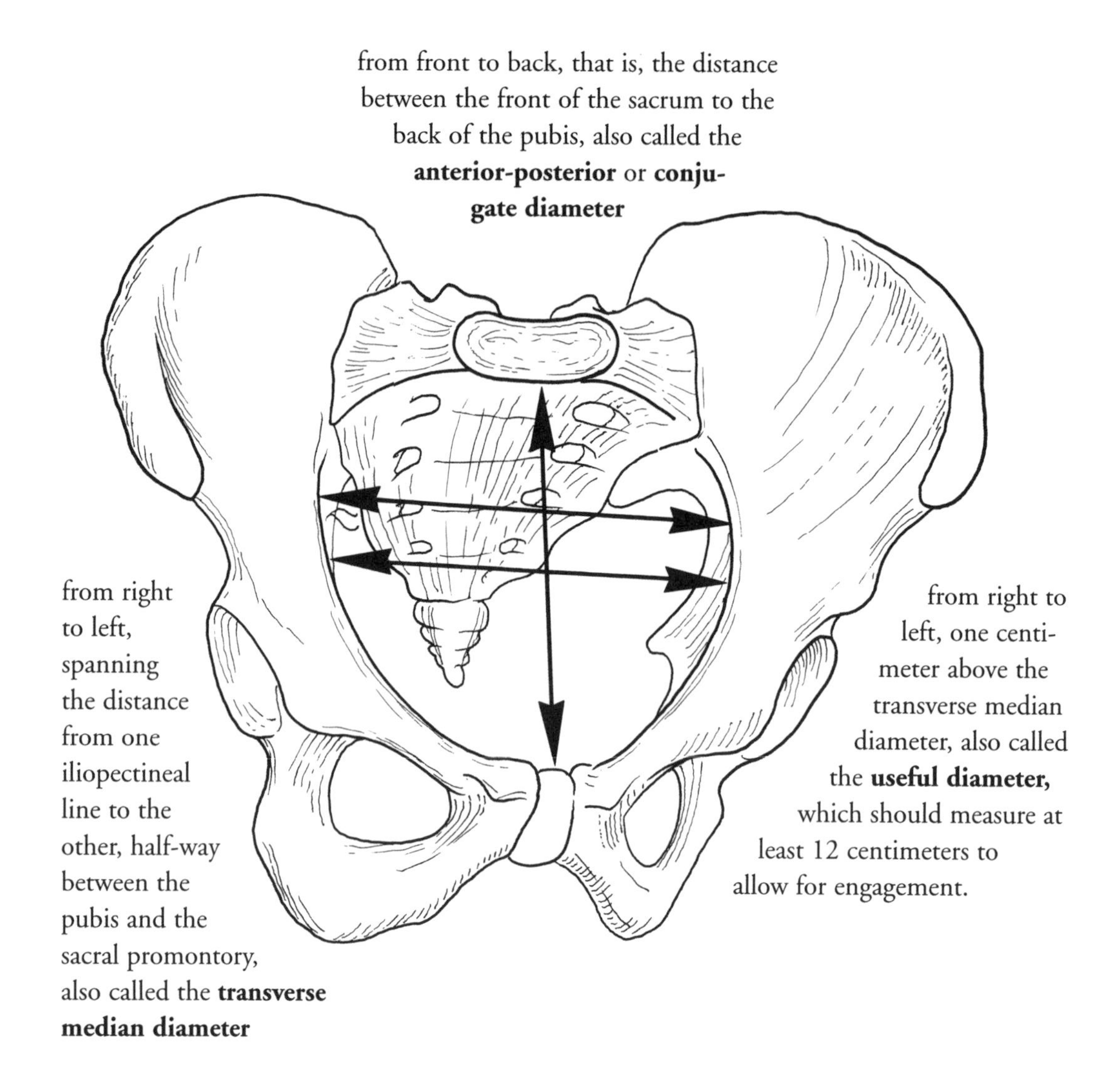

The greater the span, the more easily the child will pass through the opening. If it is small, the passage of the fetus could force apart the maternal pelvic articulations. It could also impede the passage of the child. This distance is evaluated during the final month of pregnancy or on the day of delivery, and may justify the use of a cesarean section.

The span of the superior opening is not necessarily related to the overall shape of the pelvis. Some pelvises have large iliac wings (which make the pelvis appear "big") and a small superior opening; the opposite also occurs. Similarly, the body's exterior shape is not necessarily an indication of the size of the superior opening. It would be wrong to think, for example, that a woman with "wide" hips would necessarily have a pelvis with the right dimensions for delivery.

The lesser pelvis

The superior opening demarcates two parts of the pelvis:

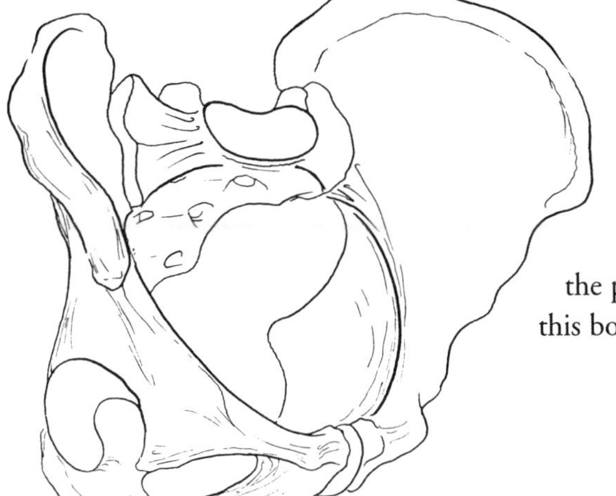

greater pelvis, which corresponds to the upper abdominal organs contained within the peritoneum,* which are not dealt with in this book

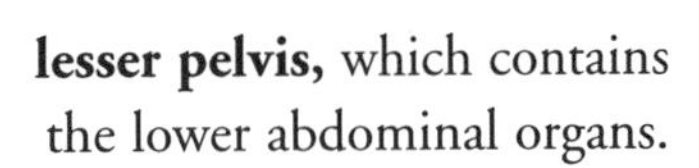

lesser pelvis, which contains the lower abdominal organs.

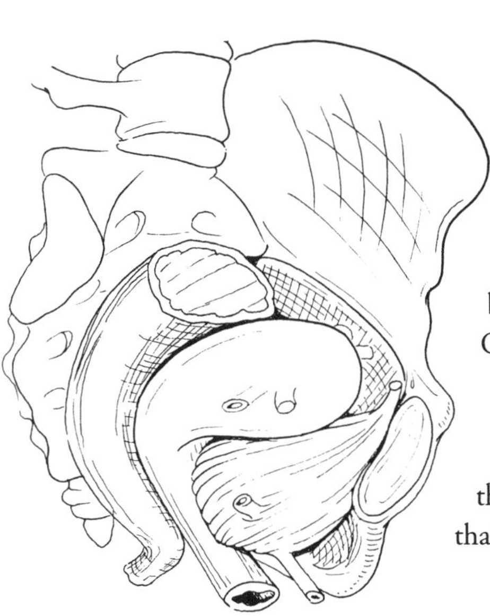

In women, the lower abdominal organs are the bladder, uterus, and rectum and are described in Chapter 3. They are also called the **subperitoneal organs** because they are below the peritoneum.

These organs are supported by what are called the **pelvic floor muscles.** These are the muscles that we will study in this book.

*The peritoneum is a serous envelope that surrounds most of the abdominal organs.

The middle opening

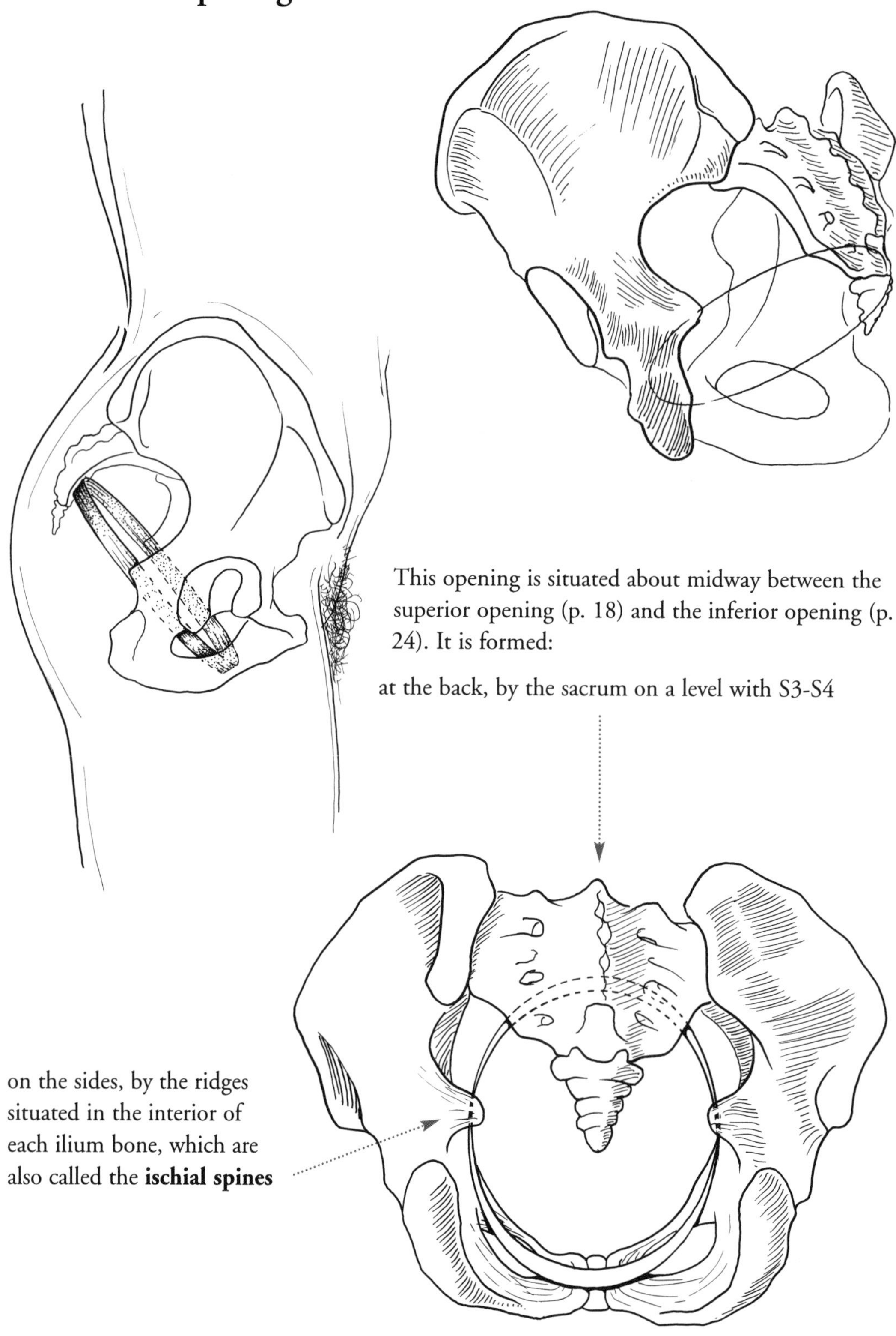

This opening is situated about midway between the superior opening (p. 18) and the inferior opening (p. 24). It is formed:

at the back, by the sacrum on a level with S3-S4

on the sides, by the ridges situated in the interior of each ilium bone, which are also called the **ischial spines**

in front, halfway up the pubic symphysis.

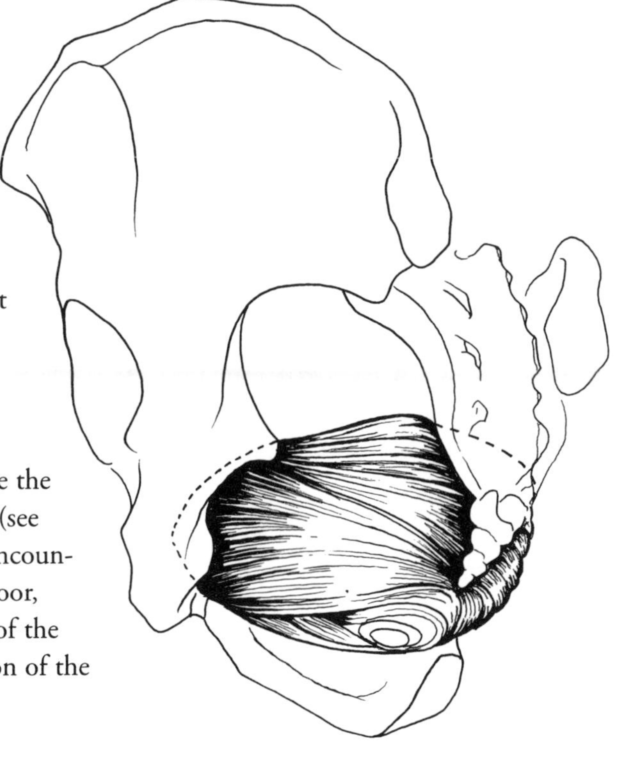

The deep muscles of the perineum, called the **pelvic diaphragm** (p. 38), are attached at the level of the middle opening. It is very important to visualize it not right at the bottom of the pelvis, but halfway up the lesser pelvis.

During delivery, the middle opening is important since the rotations that precede the final phase of the delivery are made here (see pp. 26 and 27). It is here that the head encounters the first deep muscles of the pelvic floor, which are attached to the circumference of the middle opening and will align the position of the head.

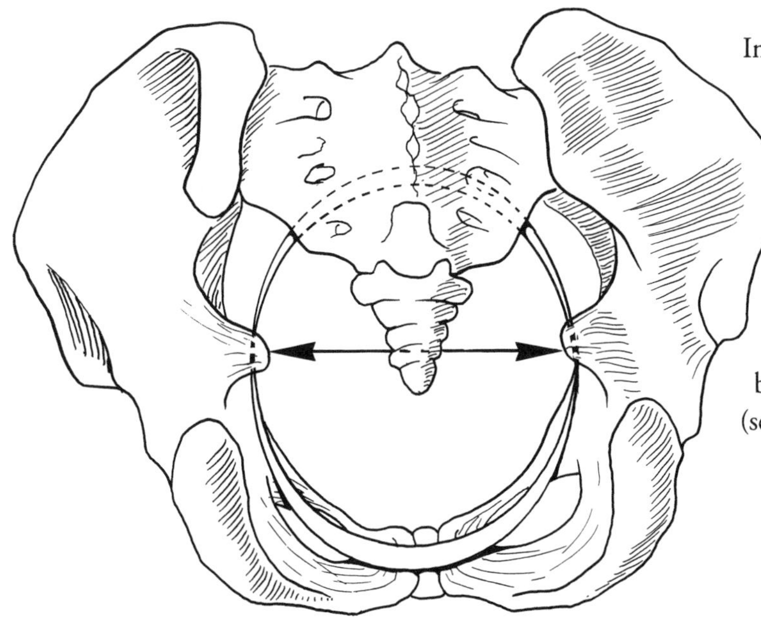

In preparation for delivery, the distance between the ischial spines is measured and is often about 10 centimeters (roughly four inches). This diameter is not to be confused with the bi-ischial diameter (see p. 24).

Note: The ishial spines can sometimes jut out too much into the interior and obstruct or even prevent a natural delivery. A cesarean section is then indicated.

The inferior opening

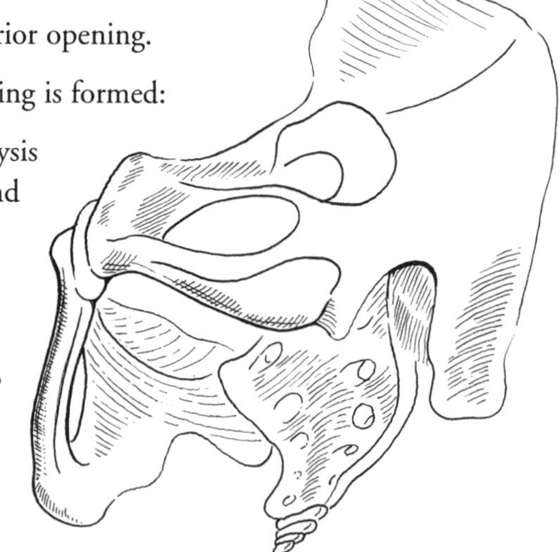

At the very bottom of the pelvic bowl is the inferior opening.

Viewing the pelvis from below, the inferior opening is formed:

- in front, by the lower edge of the pubic symphysis
- on the sides, by the lower edges of the ischia and the ischiopubic ramus (bony arches from the ischia to the pubis)
- behind, by the coccyx.

The **most superficial muscles of the perineum,** the ones closest to the skin, are attached to the inferior opening (see pp. 36 and 37).

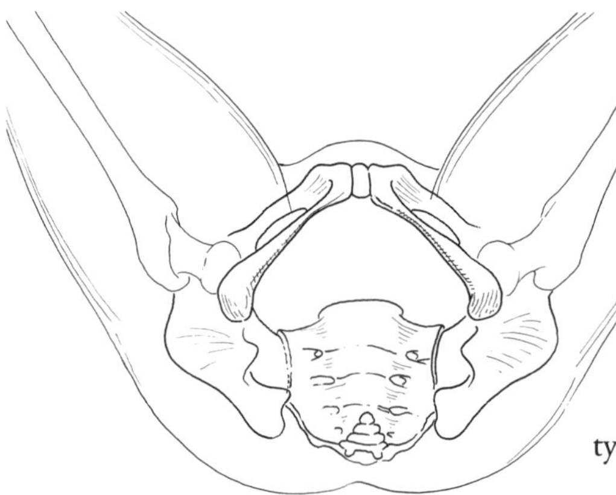

This opening is also measured for delivery, as it is the final bony passage that the fetus must transverse. Of particular importance are:

- the **bi-ischial diameter** between the two ischial tuberosities, typically 11 centimeters in length
- the distance from the pubis to the coccyx, typically from 9 to 9.5 centimeters in length.

During delivery, the coccyx can tip posteriorly. This can increase the distance from the pubis to the coccyx, which can reach 11 to 12 centimeters.

In front, the inferior opening forms an ogive (pointed arch) shape between the two ischia, the top being the pubic symphysis. Depending on its height and width, the opening can be more or less open (wide) or closed (high and narrow). The shape is important because this pubic arch is the final bony cavity that the baby must get through. This is where the baby's head first appears to the outside world. The shape of this opening is palpated during the clinical examination at nine months. If it is very closed, it could obstruct the baby's passage and justify the use of a cesarean section or forceps.

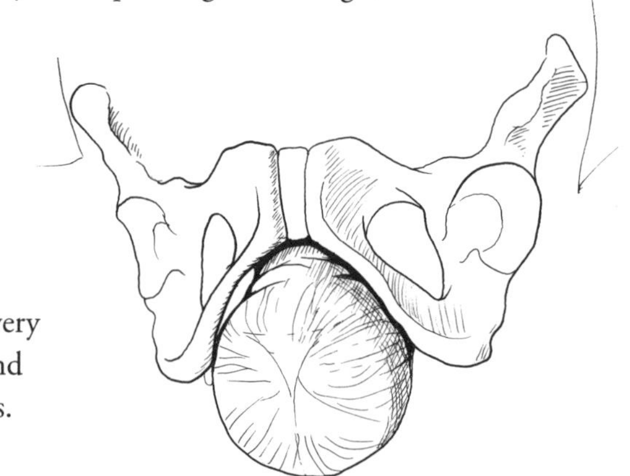

The pelvic cavity

The channel in the lesser pelvis is shaped by a succession of openings, collectively called the **pelvic cavity.**

On the day of delivery, the fetus must go through the entire bony passage. It is not a straight path, but rather a curved and fragmented tunnel.

In a woman who is upright, the superior aspect of the cavity is oblique from top to bottom and ovoid from back to front.

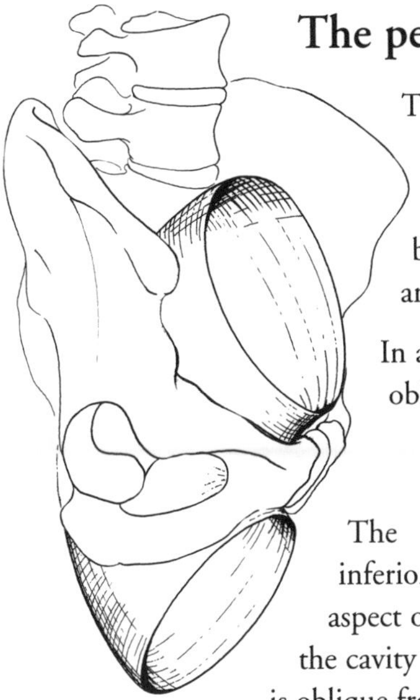

The inferior aspect of the cavity is oblique from bottom to top and ovoid from back to front.

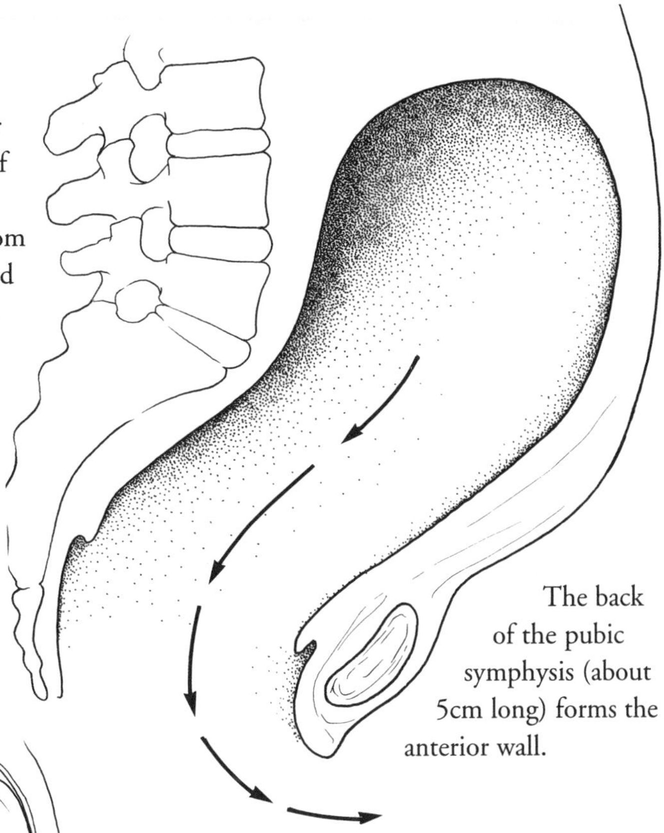

The sacrum, concave and behind, forms the cavity's posterior wall (about 16cm long).

The back of the pubic symphysis (about 5cm long) forms the anterior wall.

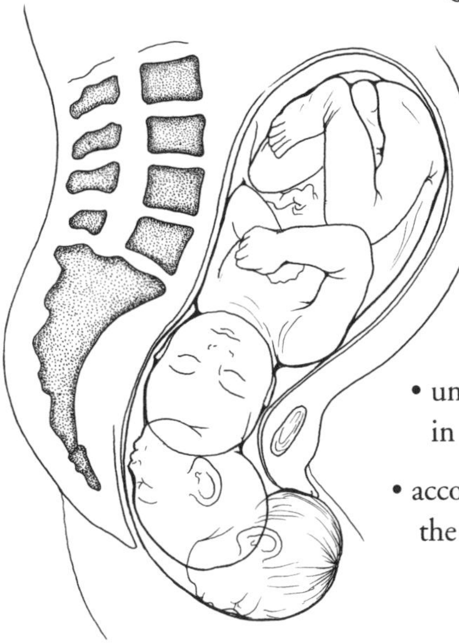

It is important to create a clear mental image of this curve to help you:

- understand the **oblique arrangement** of internal organs in the lesser pelvis
- accompany the pushing of expulsion during delivery with the maximum precision.

How the head of the fetus adapts by turning to get through the mother's pelvis

The fetal head is not spherical; it is more ovoid in shape, and therefore *has longer and shorter diameters.* It will adapt its position in order to place its shorter diameter along the longer diameters of the maternal pelvis.

As it enters the pelvis the head is still "free." The maximum diameter of the superior opening is slightly oblique from right to left (see pp. 19 and 20).

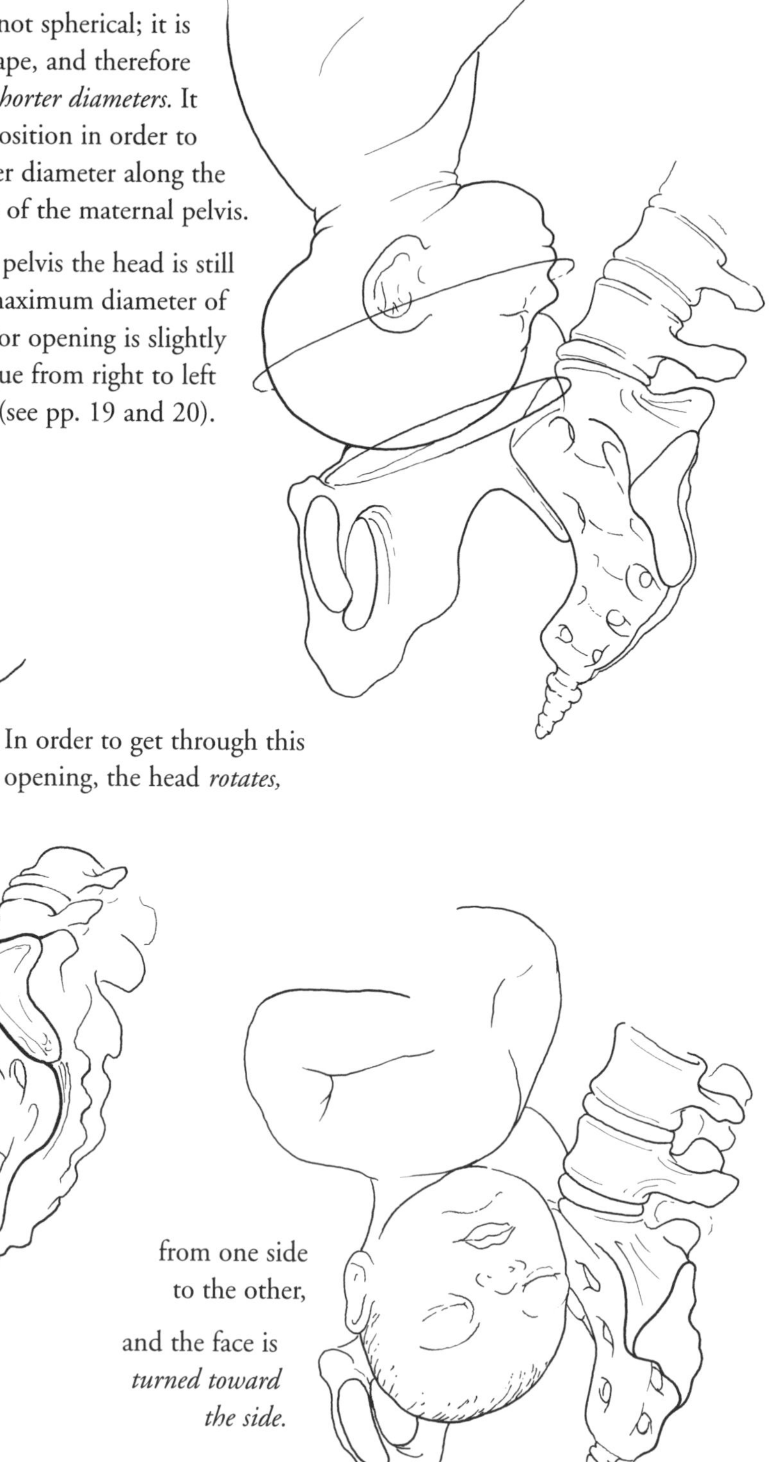

In order to get through this opening, the head *rotates,*

from one side to the other,

and the face is *turned toward the side.*

Then, as the head descends, it arrives in the middle opening. Here, between the ischial spines, the cavity is narrower from right to left (and wider from front to back).

The head *turns again a quarter turn to place the face toward the sacrum.*

Then the head bends into a *flexed position* (against the sacrum), as if to create a "double chin." This movement is an important preparatory step that will allow the fetus to present the shorter diameter of the head in the final passageway (the perineum).

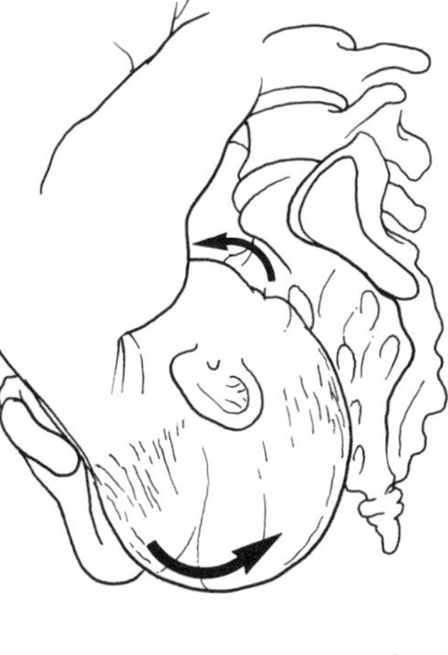

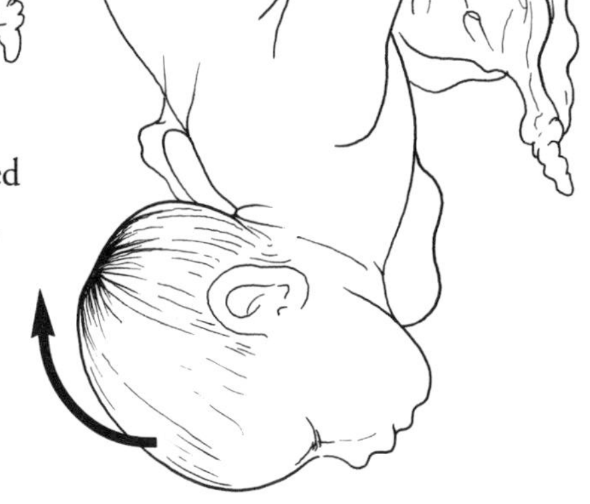

Once the head passes through this opening, it can proceed downward and find support against the pubic symphysis.

There, the head turns again, into extension. In other words, the head moves in the opposite direction when making its exit.

It's a bit like when you help dress a child and pull a sweater over the child's head. You put the neck opening over the back of the head and pull it on from back to front.

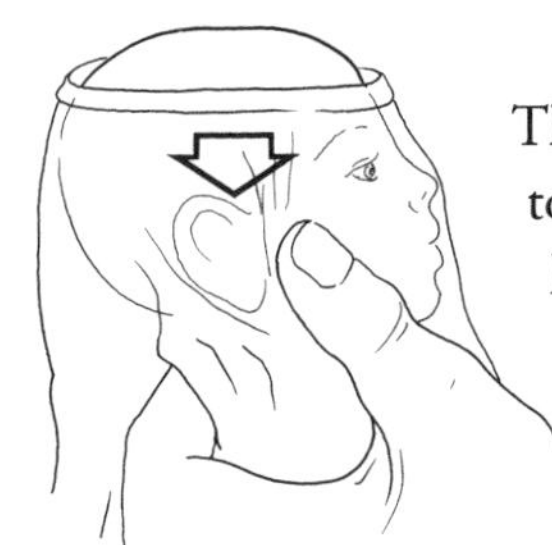

This is much easier than if you were to pull it on over the crown of the head, which is larger.

How the pelvic bones move, particularly during delivery

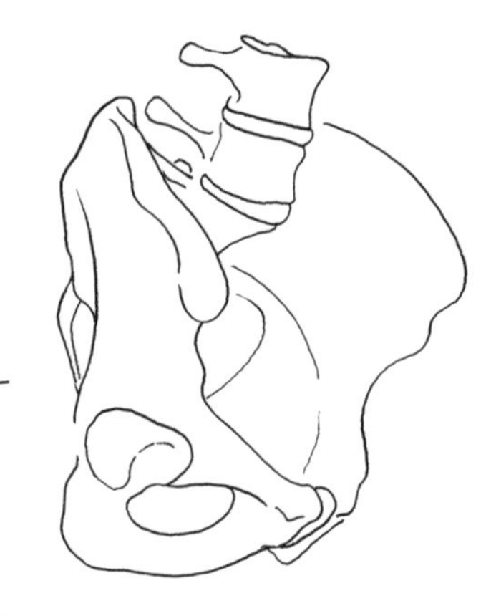

Small movements are possible between the sacrum and the ilium, simultaneously engaging the pubic symphysis and at least one sacroiliac articulation. (This is sometimes impossible in arthritic or fixed hip joints.) The movements can change both the dimensions of the pelvic openings and the shape of the cavity.

These movements are of minimal importance in everyday life, but are of maximal importance during childbirth.

The soft surfaces of the articulations absorb aqueous substances liberated by the presence of progesterone and human chorionic gonadotropin* in the blood stream, which gives them greater mobility. It is in this context that the following movements of the bones occur:

- The pubic symphysis makes very small sliding and opening movements.
- The sacroiliacs allow for a counter-nutation (see below) to accommodate the head at the point of engagement of the fetus.

As the fetus enters into the lesser pelvis (see p. 26) the diameter of the superior opening must enlarge. This movement is called **counter-nutation.** It occurs between the sacrum and ilium bones:

The base of the sacrum moves backward and the coccyx moves forward.

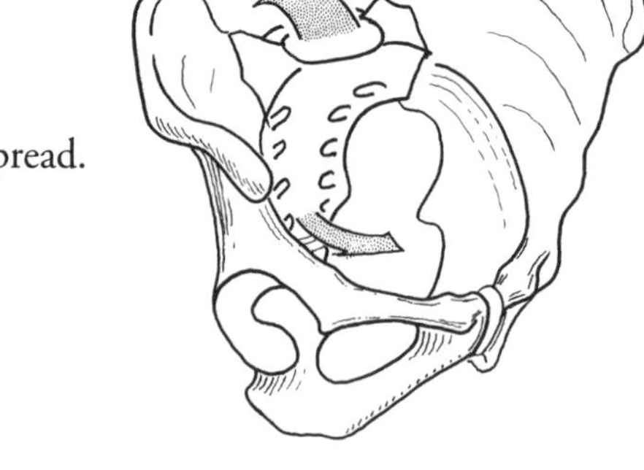

The iliac crests spread.

Concurrently, the two ischia move toward each other.

As a result of this composite movement, the diameters of the superior opening enlarge and those of the inferior opening are reduced.

*The hormone human chorionic gonadotropin increases the suppleness of the articulations.

When the fetus is engaged, the head reaches the middle opening and the other extremity of the cavity. Now the dimensions of the inferior opening must be expanded.

The movement that occurs now is called a **nutation,** the exact opposite of the preceding movement.

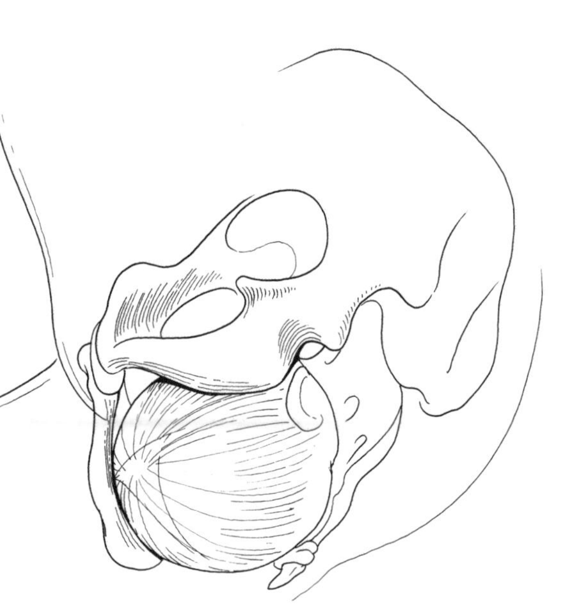

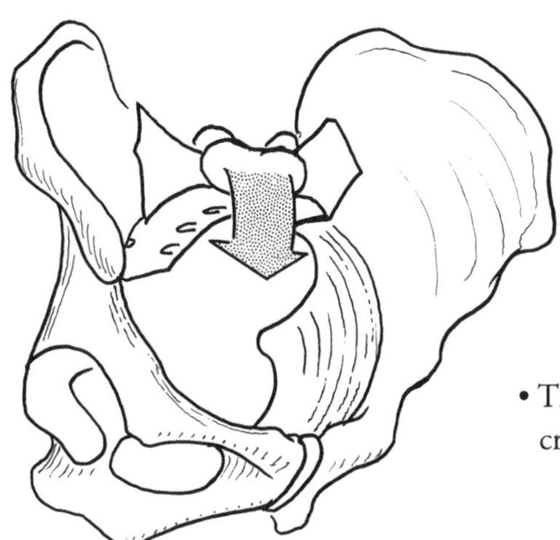

In this movement, the following occur simultaneously:

- The base of the sacrum advances, and the coccyx moves backward.
- The ischia spread apart while the iliac crests move toward each other.

As you can see in this composite movement, *the diameters of the inferior opening enlarge and those of the superior opening are reduced.*

This movement occurs during the final phase of delivery: expulsion.

In everyday life such movements occur on a very small scale. It is useful to practice them (see pp. 96-101), both to keep the pelvic bones in a state of suppleness and to exercise the muscles of the perineum.

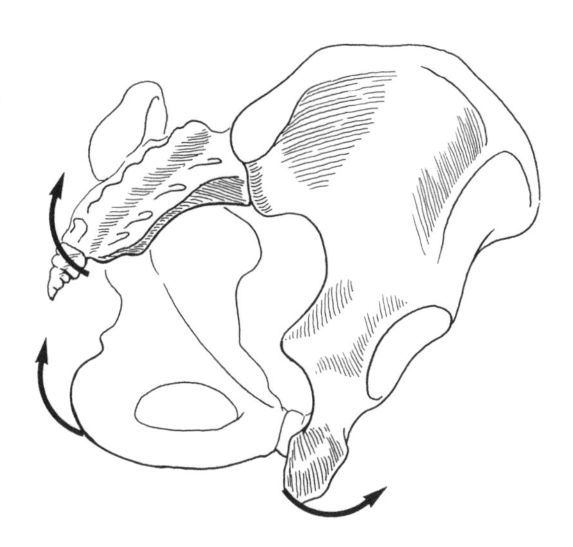

Movements that appear to be the same and are often confused...

Anterior and posterior rotation: the pelvis moves on the hip joints

The following are movements of the ilium bones upon the heads of the femur.[1] The direction of the rotations is indicated by the arrows drawn along the iliac crests. In the upright position, if the rotation tilts the pelvis forward and downward, the movement is called **anterior rotation (anteversion).**

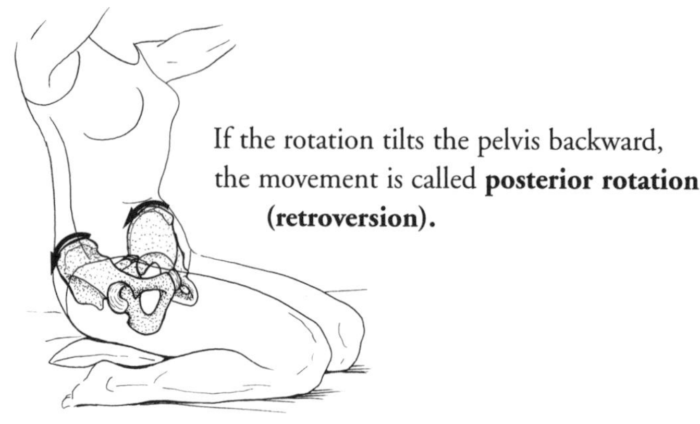

If the rotation tilts the pelvis backward, the movement is called **posterior rotation (retroversion).**

These movements are often called **pelvic rotations.**[2] They are intended to be practiced in a number of positions in preparation for childbirth:[3]

- on all fours, which is the easiest way to practice them
- lying on the back. Here, one type of rotation is easy (posterior rotation), but the other (anterior rotation) is more difficult because the pelvis is pushed against the ground.

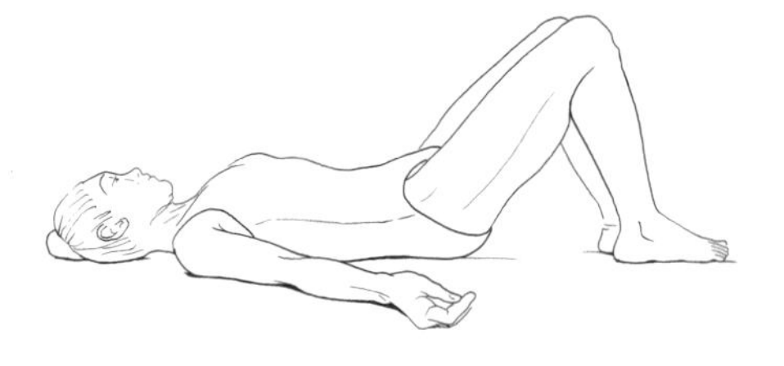

- lying on one side
- sitting on the knees (see drawings on next page).

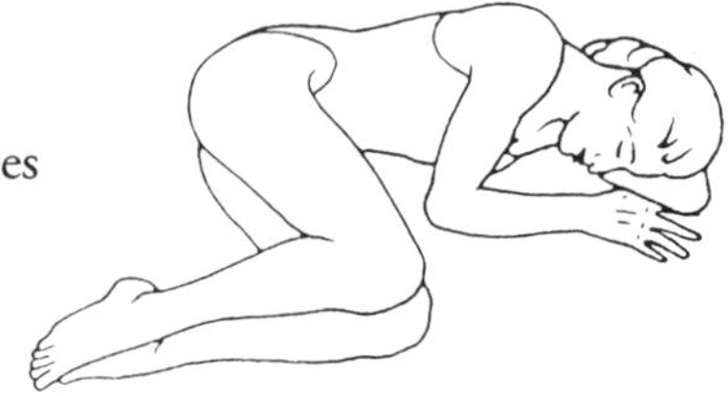

1. For the sake of simplicity, they will be described as though the pelvis rotates as one block on the hips.
2. The term *pelvic rotation* is generic as it does not indicate whether the rotation is forward or backward.
3. Making the movements described here are important during pregnancy. They mobilize the lower regions of the abdomen and activate the circulation, in particular that of the large vessels. However, they do not bring about movements between the pelvic bones, and it is precisely those movements that prepare the expecting mother for the process of delivery.

Lordosis and kyphosis: the lumbar vertebrae move back and forth

Here the vertebrae move between themselves, making a hollow shape in the lumbar region of the back.

The term **lordosis,** or "sway back," can be used to describe the normal curvature of the back, also known as the **lumbar curve.**

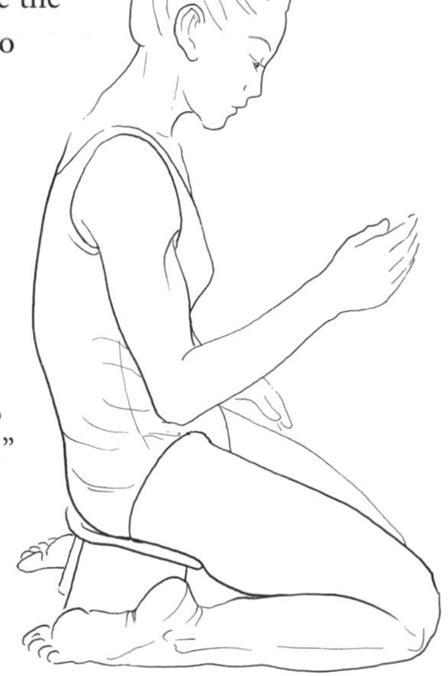

Alternatively, the vertebrae move in the opposite direction to round the back, a process called **kyphosis,** or "round back."

These movements resemble those described on the previous page, except that those described here occur a little higher in the lumbar curve, up near the waist.

To understand the perineum, it is important to distinguish between and have an accurate idea of the sensations and actions that originate in this region.

During pregnancy, the baby's weight and the greater suppleness of the articulations accentuate anteversion and lordosis and carry the abdomen forward. There is no need to be alarmed by this unless the changes cause pain, in which case you can try the exercises on pp. 102 and 103.

The two triangles of the perineum

If you look at the bony pelvis from below you will see four bony protrusions: the pubis, the coccyx, and the two ischial tuberosities, which together make up the four corners of the diamond-shaped **perineum.**

The perineum (or "pelvic floor") is divided into two triangles by a line joining the two tuberosities. This line is formed by the two superficial transverse perineal muscles (p. 36).

The anterior perineum corresponds to the anterior triangle, which corresponds to the urogenital space. The orifices of the vagina and the urethra are located within this space.

The posterior perineum corresponds to the posterior triangle, which corresponds to the rectal space. The terminal orifice of the anus is found within this space.

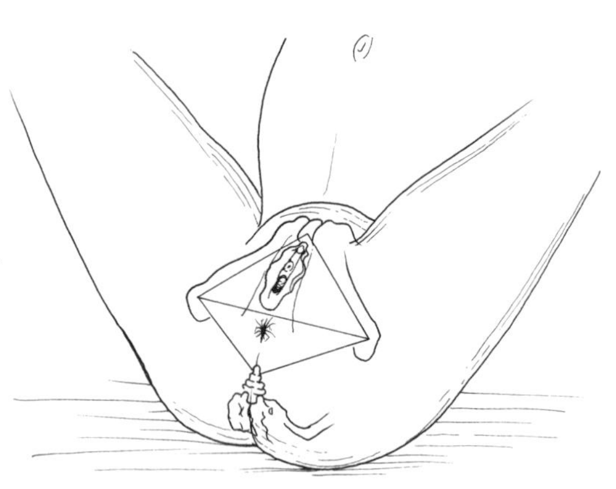

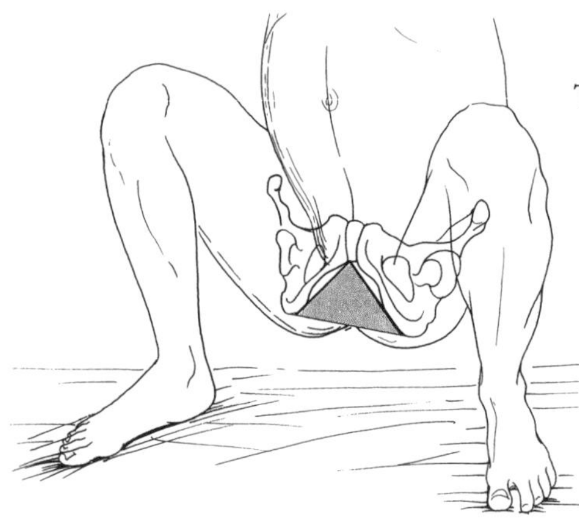

The anterior triangle is oblique forward and downward.

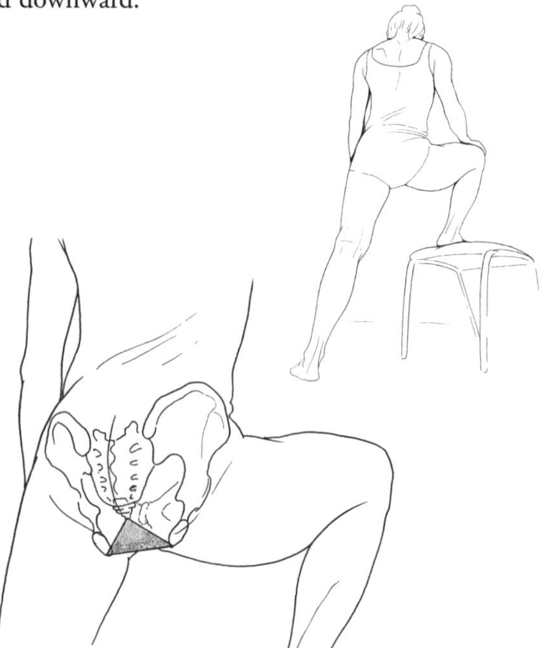

The posterior triangle is oblique backward and downward.

External morphology: the pelvic bones and the external female genitals

The anterior triangle is delineated on its sides by the ischiopubic rami and in front by the pubic symphysis. There we find a zone covered by hair, called the **mons pubis.**

The **labia minora** are the two thin, irregularly-edged cutaneous folds. Here they are shown spread out, but usually they are stuck together. In front, they double up to form the hood of the **clitoris** (p. 37).

The posterior triangle is delineated by the two ischial tuberosities and the coccyx.

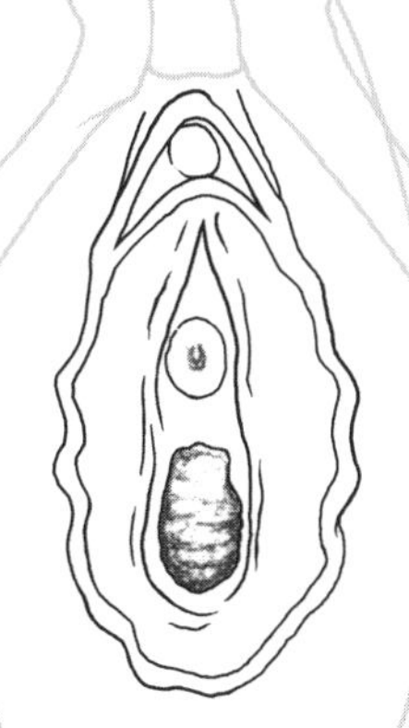

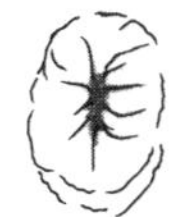

Next are the large **labia majora,** which are the folds bordering each side from front to back. The **vulva** is the zone common to the structures of both the urethra and the vagina.

The **anus** is situated behind the vulva to which it is connected by a fibrous, muscular area known as the **central tendon** of the perineum or perineal body (p. 42).

pelvis viewed from below

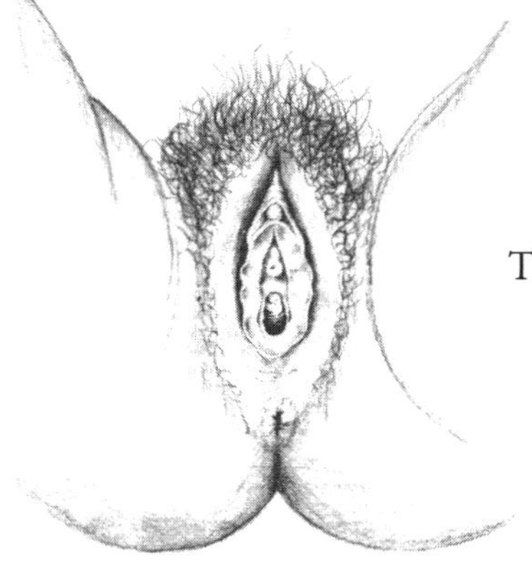

The erectile bodies are described on p. 37.

CHAPTER TWO

The Musculature of the Perineum

Having familiarized ourselves with the bony pelvis, we will now study the muscles that make up the perineum. In other words, we will look at those parts of the perineum that can contract and expand, and those that are stretched passively because of their elasticity.

The perineum consists of two types of muscles:

The **muscles of the pelvic floor** will be studied in this chapter. They are a collection of muscles that effectively form a floor, and are arranged in two main layers: a superficial and a deep layer. This assemblage of muscles supports and holds up the organs of the lower pelvis (bladder, uterus, and rectum).

There are also **muscles associated with the orifices** of the pelvic organs: the sphincters of the urethra and anus, the muscles of the rectum, and the column of the vagina. These are much smaller than the muscles that make up the pelvic floor. They will be studied in Chapter 4 in connection with the abdominal organs.

These two types of muscles are fairly intertwined, with adhesions and crisscrossed fibrous layers. However, in order to create a clear and precise mental picture of the area, it is important to distinguish between them. This will be of great help in determining the proper sensations and muscular actions that each of them should have. Otherwise there will be much confusion.

The pelvic floor

This is the name given to the group of muscles that encloses the bottom of the lower pelvis. It is composed of two layers:

- a superficial layer of long fibrous muscles that is called the **perineum** (associated with the layer of skin above it)
- a deep layer of large thick muscles, also called the **pelvic diaphragm.**

This assemblage of muscles is inserted into the internal surface of the lesser pelvis, the deep layer around the rim of the middle opening, and the superficial layer around the inferior rim (or opening). Several useful observations can be made about these muscles:

- The fibers are oriented downward and outward.
- The whole group is shaped like the hull of a boat.
- The muscles cross over each other and surround the three orifices (or apertures): the urethra, vagina, and anus (contributing to sphincter control).

This muscular structure serves a dual function:

- *It supports the lower abdomen.* This support is increased during the effort of childbirth and when there is an increase in the volume and weight of the internal organs. This function is particularly attributable to the contractile quality of the muscles.
- *It serves as a passageway from the interior to the exterior,* a feat which can be attributed to the elasticity of the musculature.

The superficial layer of perineal muscles

These muscles form a structure from front to back between the pubis and the coccyx and laterally between the two ischial tuberosities.

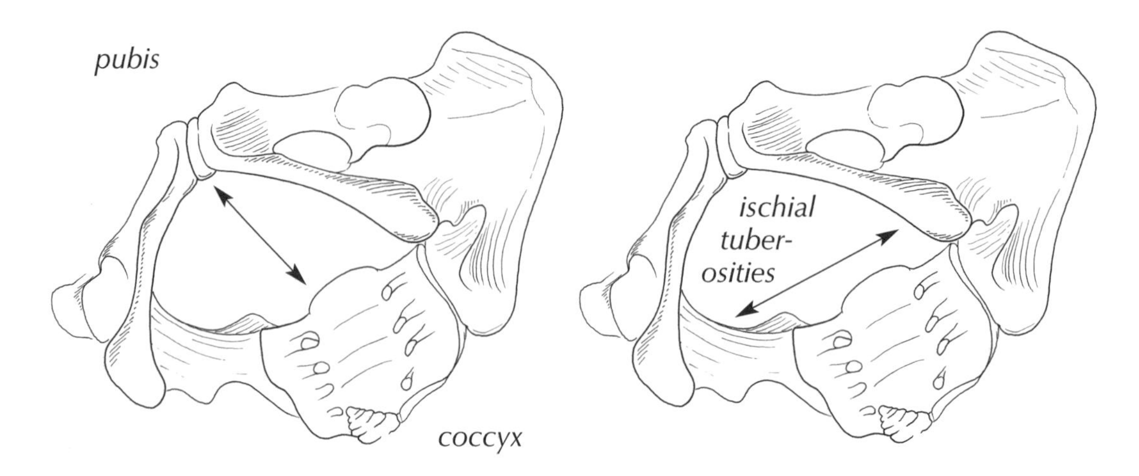

The muscles form a figure 8 that crosses over at a zone called the central tendinous point of the perineum, or simply, the **central tendon**. In front, the anterior loop of this figure 8 is situated within a triangle of muscles (see p. 37).

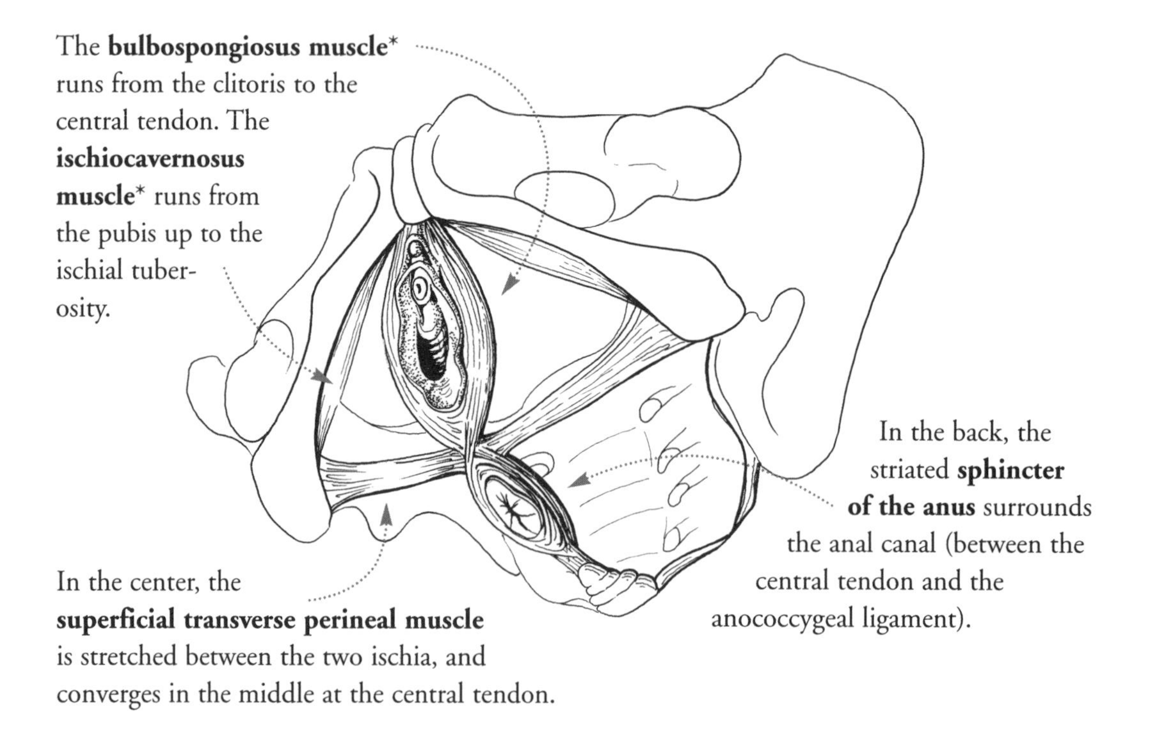

The **bulbospongiosus muscle*** runs from the clitoris to the central tendon. The **ischiocavernosus muscle*** runs from the pubis up to the ischial tuberosity.

In the back, the striated **sphincter of the anus** surrounds the anal canal (between the central tendon and the anococcygeal ligament).

In the center, the **superficial transverse perineal muscle** is stretched between the two ischia, and converges in the middle at the central tendon.

*The bulbospongiosus and ischiocavernosus muscles cover the erectile bodies (see next page).

An overview of the muscles of the superficial layer of the perineum

Two sets of muscles are situated in the anterior triangle and are often included in a description of the superficial layer. They are found between the layers of a double-layered partition called the **perineal membrane**.

The **external sphincter of the urethra** surrounds the lowest part of the urethra.

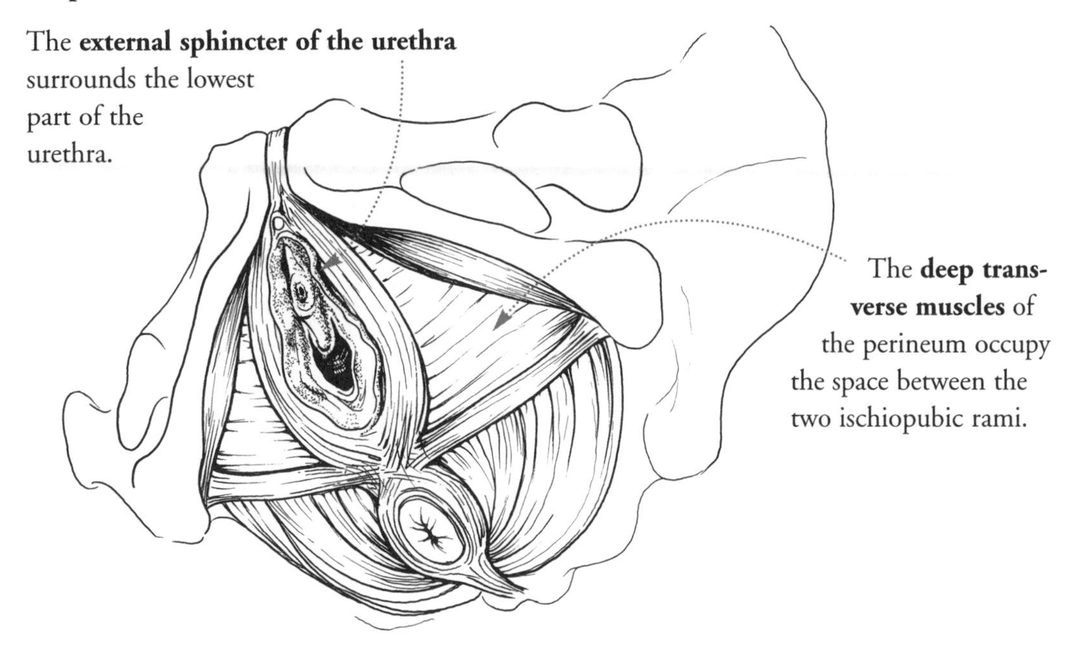

The **deep transverse muscles** of the perineum occupy the space between the two ischiopubic rami.

The **erectile bodies** are fixed beneath the deep layer of the membrane. These are organs formed of tissue rich in capillaries, which can dilate and swell.

The **corpus cavernosum** runs along each ischiopubic ramus and joins at the front to create the body of the clitoris.

The **clitoris** is the erectile body analagous to the male penis. It is situated just behind the pubis. It is cylindrical in shape and is about three centimeters long and half a centimeter in diameter.

The **vestibular bulbs** are situated on each side of the vulva.

The **Bartholin's glands** are located behind the posterior part of the vulva. They secrete a lubricating substance that flows into the vagina during sexual intercourse.

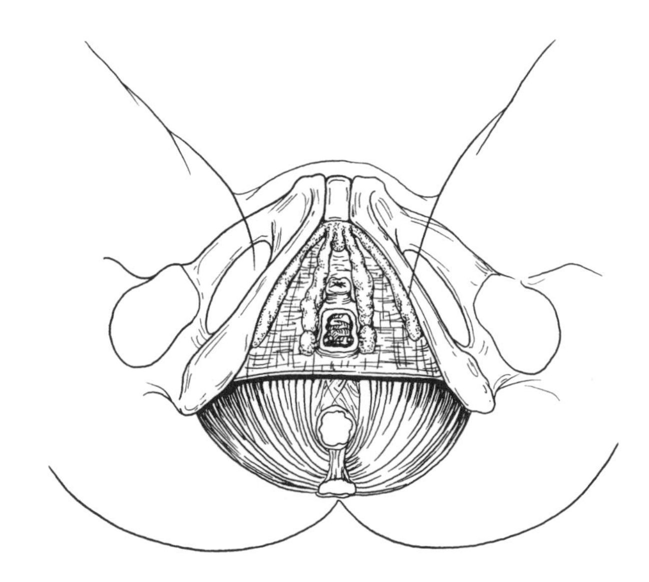

The deep layer of the pelvic muscles

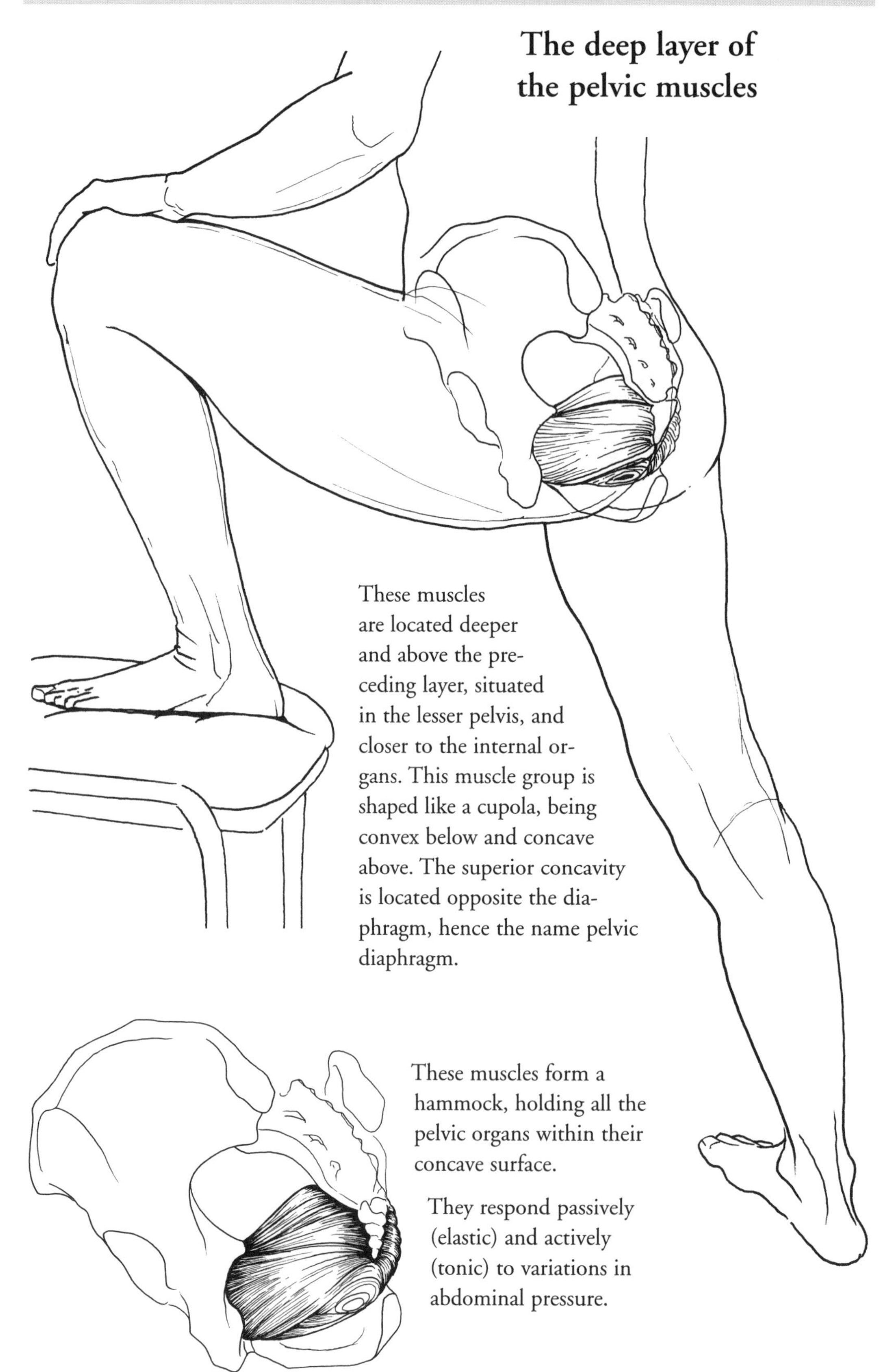

These muscles are located deeper and above the preceding layer, situated in the lesser pelvis, and closer to the internal organs. This muscle group is shaped like a cupola, being convex below and concave above. The superior concavity is located opposite the diaphragm, hence the name pelvic diaphragm.

These muscles form a hammock, holding all the pelvic organs within their concave surface.

They respond passively (elastic) and actively (tonic) to variations in abdominal pressure.

Here we find two muscles:

The **levator ani** is a powerful muscle made up of different bundles of muscles arranged around the apertures of the internal organs. It is horseshoe-shaped and consistes of two main parts:

- A medial part composed of the **puborectalis muscle,** which begins above the pubis and slings around the rectum, and the adjacent **pubococcygeus muscle,** which reaches from the tendinous arc on the ischium and surrounds the rectum.
- A lateral part called the **ilio-coccygeus muscle,** com-posed of a large sheet of fibrous bundles that begins along the pos-terior tendinous arc and ends at the coccyx.

These bundles of muscle fibers are very important for the support of the internal organs (see p. 116).

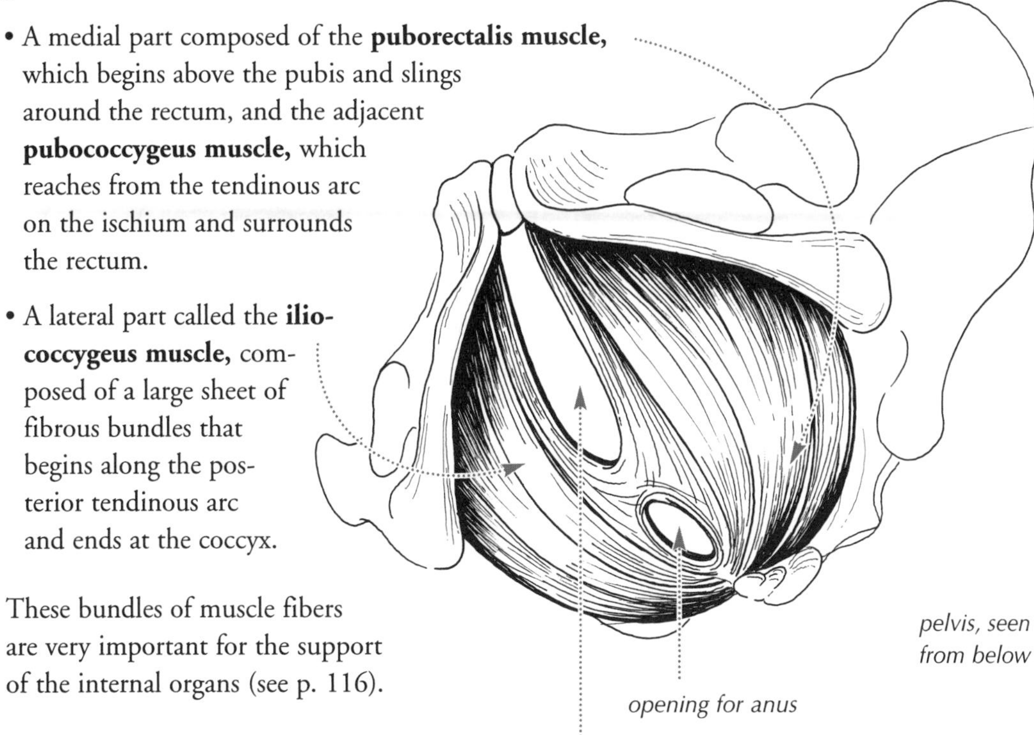

pelvis, seen from below

The **coccygeus muscle** is located behind and on the same level as the levator ani. This muscle is stretched between the ischial spine, sacrum, and coccyx.

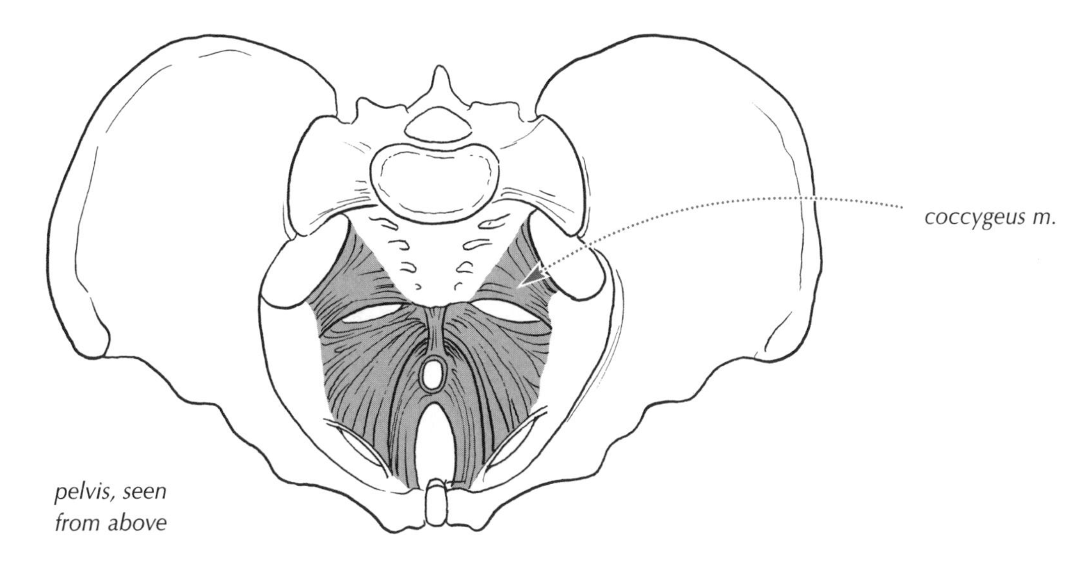

pelvis, seen from above

The urogenital hiatus

At the front, the insertion of the levator ani muscles on the right and left form an indentation or groove, a zone free of muscles that is sometimes called the **levator buttonhole** or **urogenital hiatus**.

This zone corresponds to the junction of the bladder/urethra and of the uterus/vagina.

It is at one and the same time a *wide passageway for childbearing* and *the weak spot in the supporting structure* (see p 49).

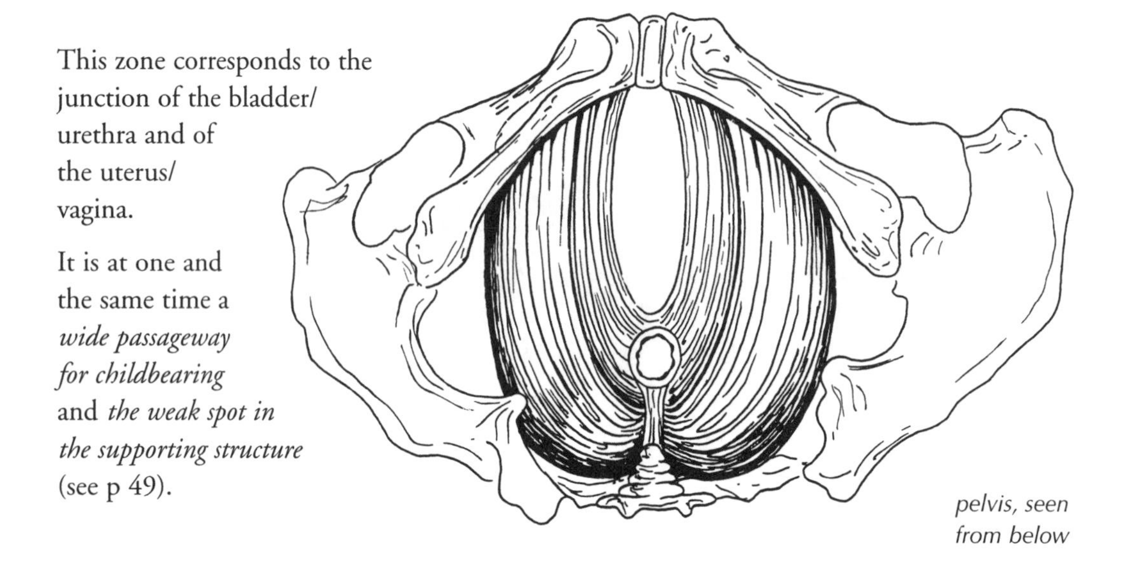

pelvis, seen from below

It is very important that the most median muscles of the levator ani (the puborectalis bundle) have good tone in order to actively support the internal organs of this region (the bladder and uterus).

Weakness of this muscle is almost always the cause of prolapse or incontinence.

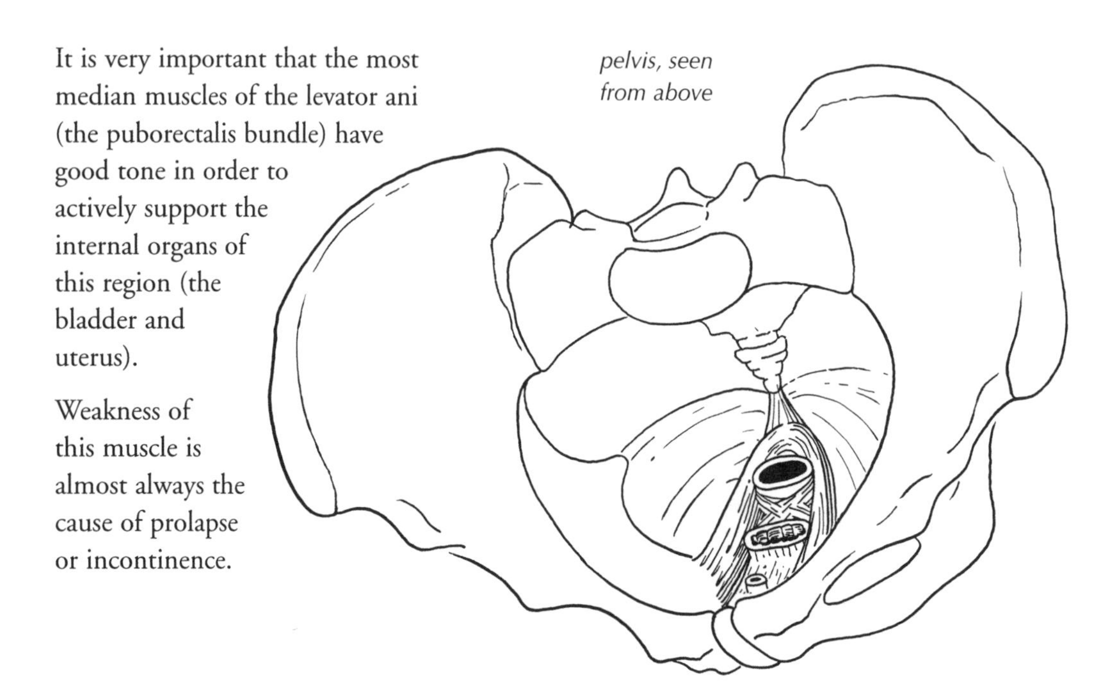

pelvis, seen from above

The two levels of the pelvic floor muscles

The two layers of muscles described in the preceding pages—the superficial and deep layers—are situated at different levels in the lesser pelvis. They also have different shapes and orientations.

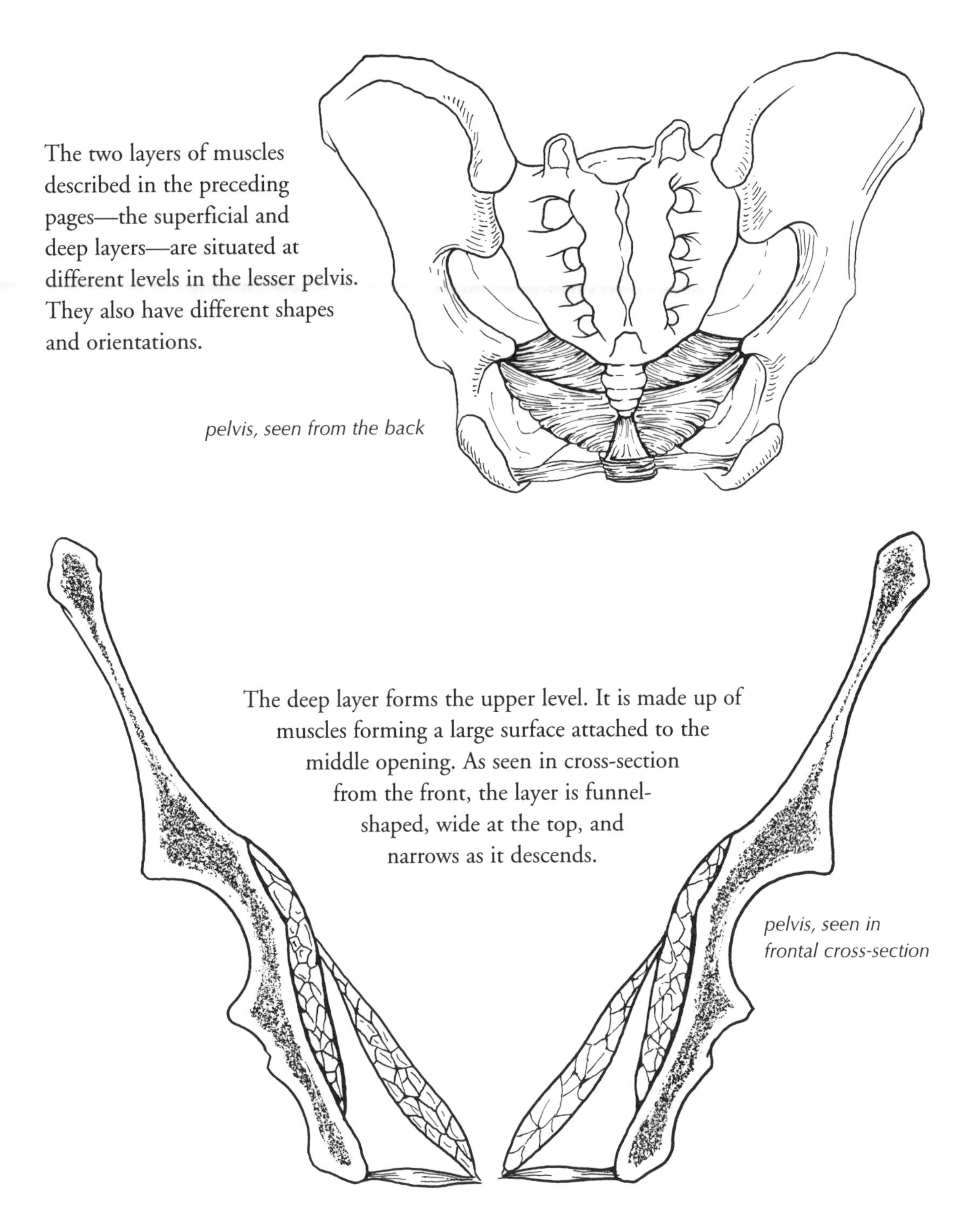

pelvis, seen from the back

The deep layer forms the upper level. It is made up of muscles forming a large surface attached to the middle opening. As seen in cross-section from the front, the layer is funnel-shaped, wide at the top, and narrows as it descends.

pelvis, seen in frontal cross-section

The superficial layer forms the lower level. It is made up of thin, interlaced bundles of muscle attached to the inferior opening. As seen in cross-section from the front, this layer is horizontal.

Where the muscles cross we find:

The central tendon of the perineum

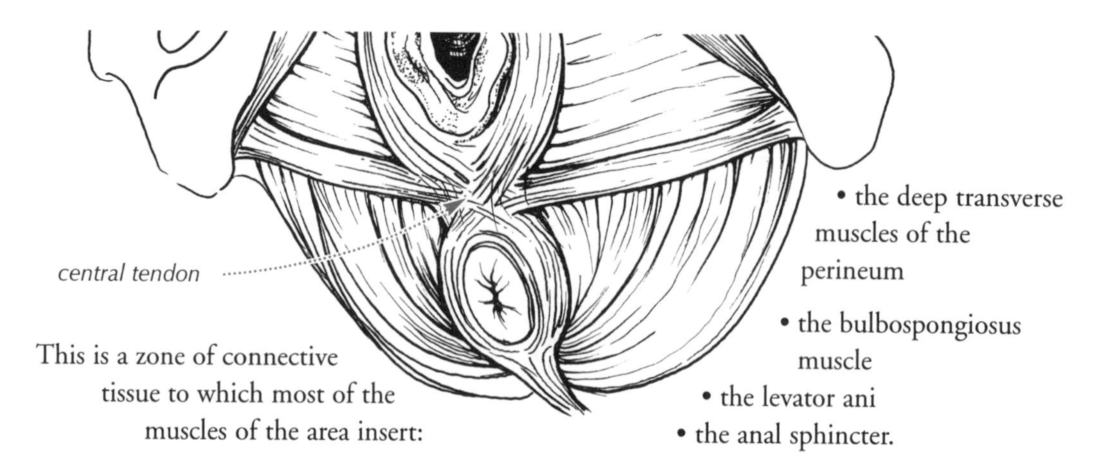

This is a zone of connective tissue to which most of the muscles of the area insert:

- the deep transverse muscles of the perineum
- the bulbospongiosus muscle
- the levator ani
- the anal sphincter.

The central tendon is very resilient. It is situated at the center of the surrounding structure and serves as an anchoring point for the surrounding musculature.

The central tendon and childbirth

This area is put under pressure during childbirth, particularly at the moment the head engages. In order to protect it from tearing, the pushing or bearing-down action is suspended to allow for its gradual expansion.

Episiotomy

A surgical procedure called **episiotomy** is sometimes performed in this area. It can be done when the thickened perineum is under pressure to release the fetus, or later when the expanded perineum is unnaturally thin with a risk of tearing.

An episiotomy can protect the central tendon if it is performed correctly, that is, before the tissues become white (the sign of an interruption of the microvasculature). Afterward, the suturing process is of utmost importance. Each section must be sutured one after the other, and any event, such as microhemorrhages, must be completely taken care of. This is vital to good postnatal function of the perineum. The performance of certain exercises during pregnancy and childbirth can reduce the need for an episiotomy (see pp. 139-143).

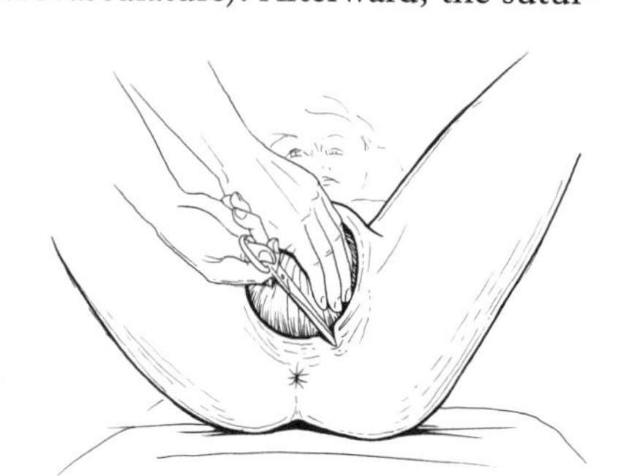

CHAPTER THREE

The Organs of the Lesser Pelvis

The bladder, uterus, and rectum are all situated in the lowest and most restricted part of the pelvis: the **pelvic bowl**. Each of the these organs belongs to a different system:

- the bladder to the urinary system
- the uterus to the reproductive system
- the rectum to the digestive system.

Each organ has an orifice that extends through the muscles of the pelvic floor, which provides an aponeurotic support system. Each organ has contractile and elastic muscles, which ensure proper filling and emptying, as needed. Great mobility is required to cope with the positional shifts caused by changes in volume in the three organs. As the interior of the pelvis itself is relatively rigid, movement occurs in the musculo-ligamentous tissues surrounding the organs.

In this chapter we will discuss the arrangement of each of these organs, as well as the systems that hold them in position in the lower pelvis. In order to exercise each part of this region with precision, it is important to form a clear mental picture of the structures, both the organs themselves and their supporting elements. To that end, only the described structures are shown in the accompanying illustrations.

General arrangement of the organs of the pelvic bowl

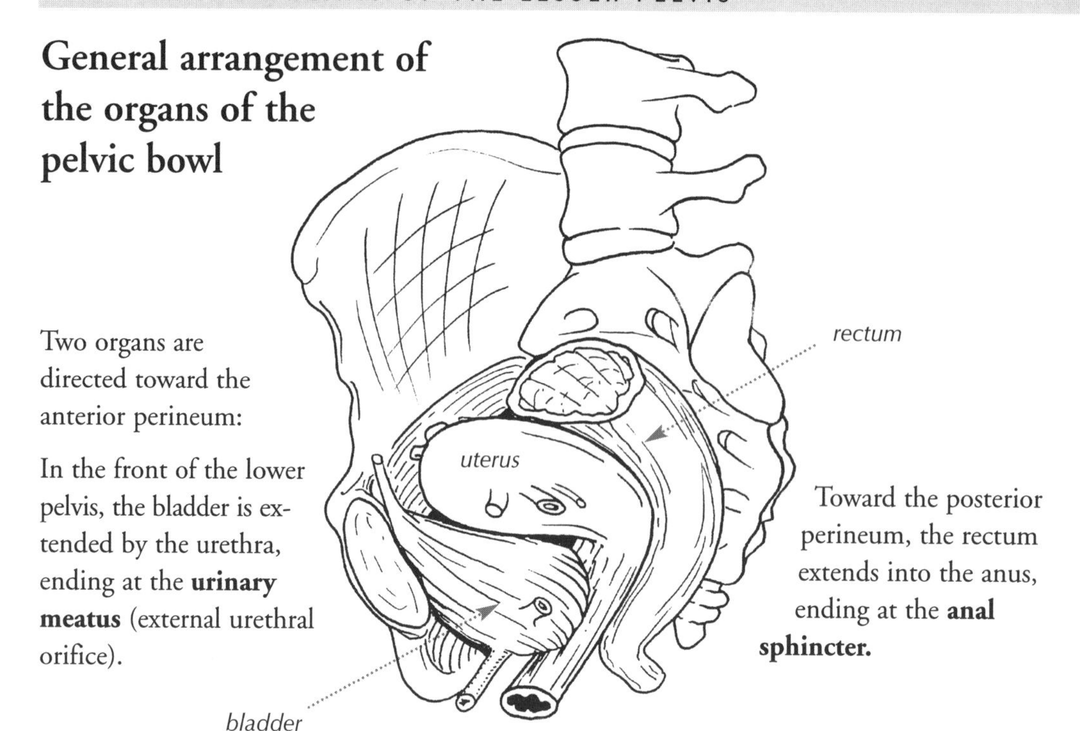

Two organs are directed toward the anterior perineum:

In the front of the lower pelvis, the bladder is extended by the urethra, ending at the **urinary meatus** (external urethral orifice).

Toward the posterior perineum, the rectum extends into the anus, ending at the **anal sphincter.**

The uterus extends into the cervix and reaches its lower opening, the **vaginal orifice,** through the vaginal canal.

These organs seemingly fold one against the other. The rectum rests against the coccyx and the posterior of the levator ani, the uterus against the bladder, and the bladder against the vagina.

This "overlapping" arrangement lends stability to the organs, especially in the upright position.

However, this stability can be compromised by abnormal positioning of one of the organs, e.g., posterior rotation of the uterus.

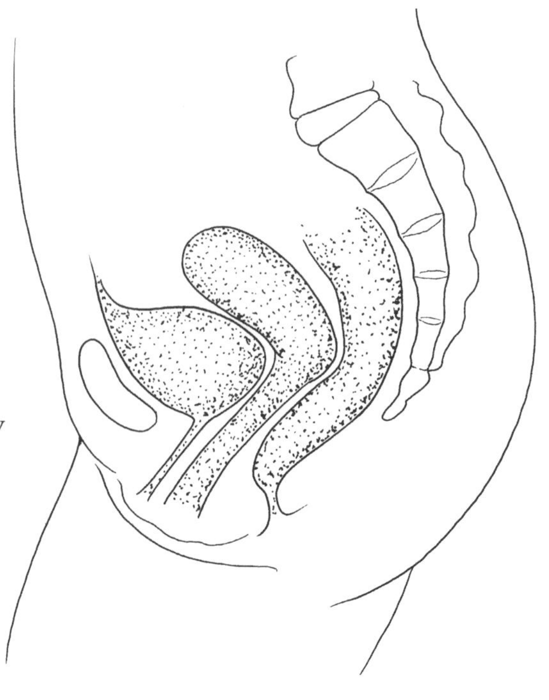

The pelvic organs are held in place by several mechanisms

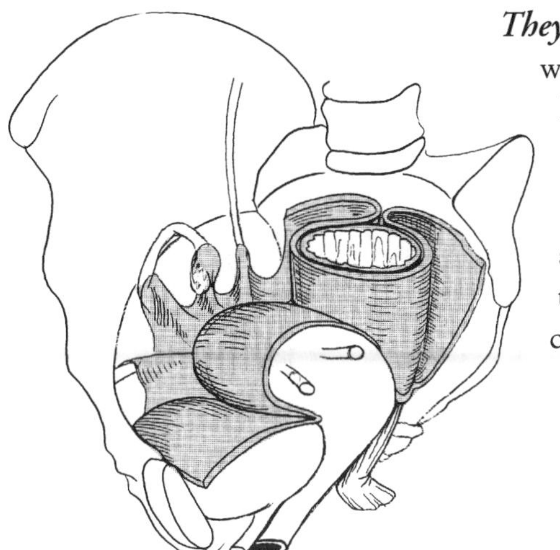

They fit against each other. This arrangement, whereby the organs fold over each other, helps to hold them together (see preceding page).

They are held up and partitioned. The organs are held up by, and adhere strongly to, the inferior section of the peritoneum, which closely covers their surfaces, forming two pouches: the vesicouterine pouch and the rectouterine pouch.

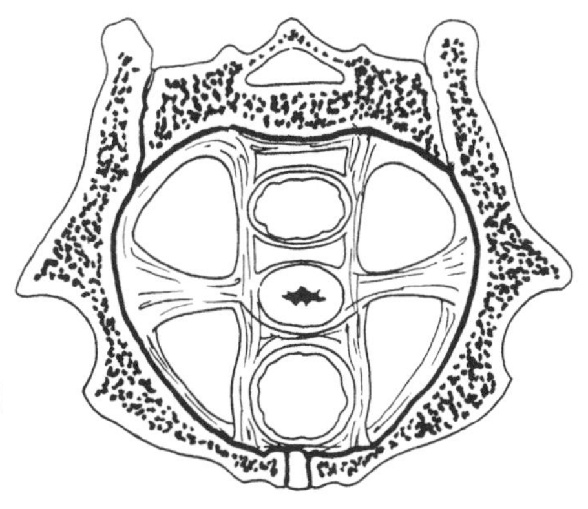

Partitioning can occur in two different directions:

- *Lateral partitioning.* On each side of the uterus, the peritoneal layer forms a large fold, held up by the fallopian tubes, called the broad ligament (see p. 56).
- *Partitioning from front to back.* The three organs are bordered on each side by two fibrous bands that stretch from the sacrum to the pubis: the sacro-genital folds. They are less important at the front.

They adhere to each other. Certain parts of these organs are joined together in places, e.g., the vagina and the urethra adhere to each other by fascial tissue.

They are supported from below by the muscles of the pelvic floor (see Chapter 2). This is an active structure that can contract or stretch, unlike the mechanisms previously described.

There are a number of factors that stabilize the organs, in different ways, while allowing them to sometimes change their volumes considerably. If some of these structures are damaged, particularly during the final phase of delivery, the overall internal balance can be disturbed.

The bladder

The bladder is a muscular membranous sac where urine accumulates between urinations.

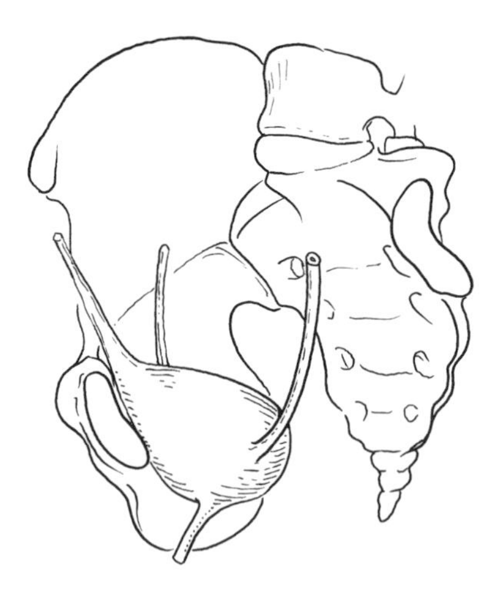

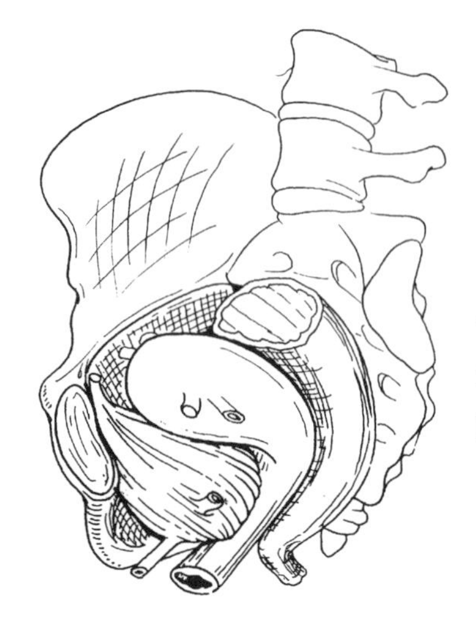

The bladder is the most forward of the organs in the lower pelvis, situated just behind the pubis, and in front of the uterus.

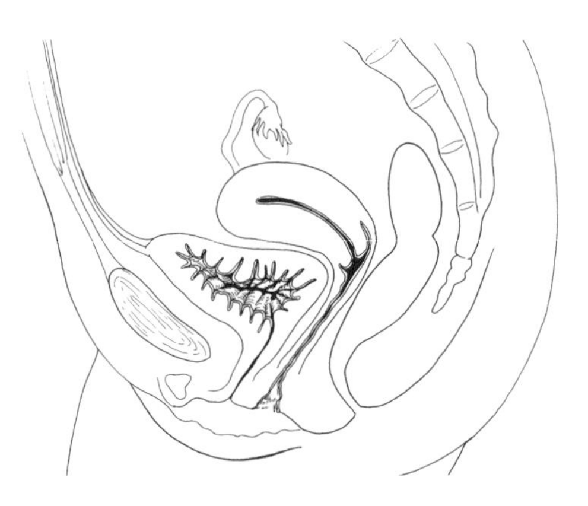

The form and volume of the bladder changes a great deal. When it is empty, it is small and folds back on itself, without rising above the pubis. (At this stage, it contains only a few milliliters of urine.) In addition, its internal surface has numerous folds.

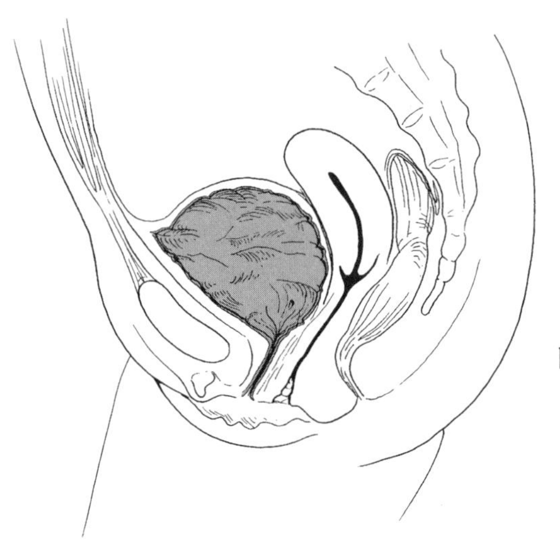

By contrast, when it is full (containing on average from 500 milliliters up to 2 liters of urine), it dilates. It becomes spherical in shape and pushes upward into the abdomen. In addition, the internal surface unfolds and becomes smooth.

Urine flows drop by drop via the two ureters from the kidneys into the bladder.

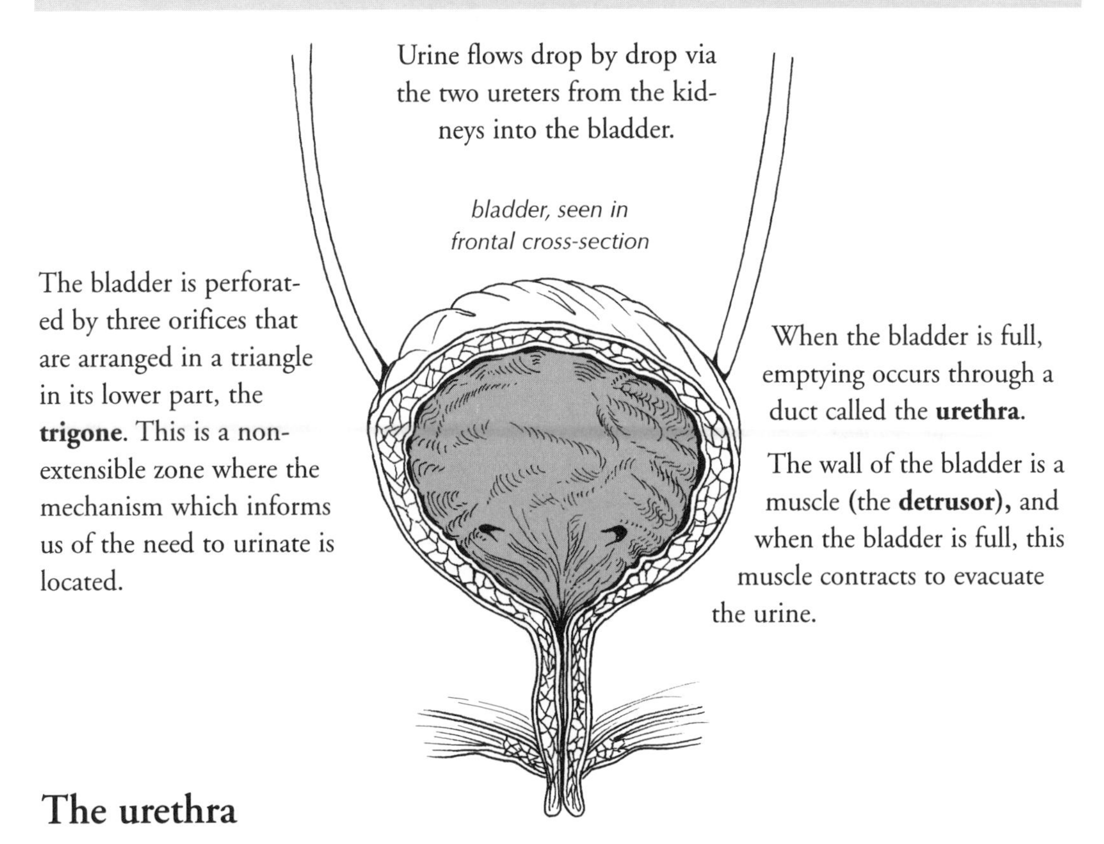

The bladder is perforated by three orifices that are arranged in a triangle in its lower part, the **trigone**. This is a nonextensible zone where the mechanism which informs us of the need to urinate is located.

When the bladder is full, emptying occurs through a duct called the **urethra**.

The wall of the bladder is a muscle (the **detrusor**), and when the bladder is full, this muscle contracts to evacuate the urine.

The urethra

The urethra is the duct through which urine accumulated in the bladder is passed to the exterior.

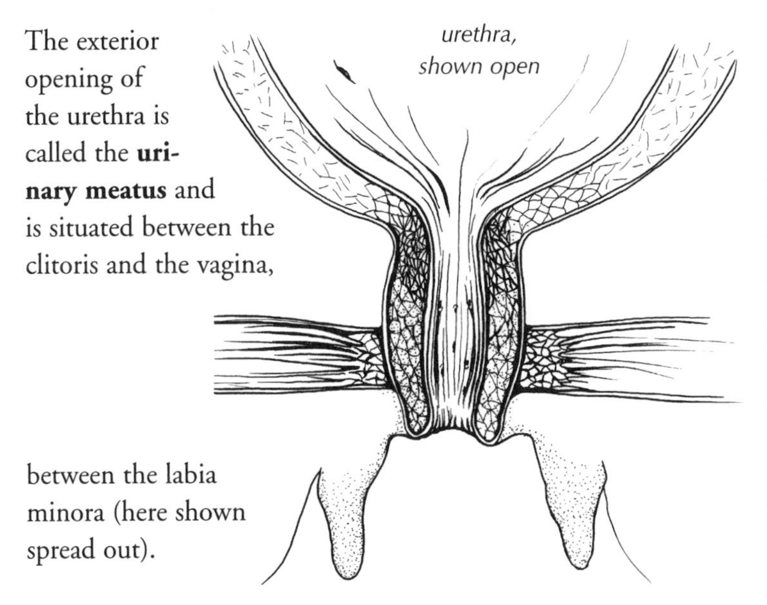

The exterior opening of the urethra is called the **urinary meatus** and is situated between the clitoris and the vagina, between the labia minora (here shown spread out).

The sphincter muscle can tighten the urethra. The **internal sphincter** is at the highest point closest to the bladder. It is a reflex involuntary muscle, i.e., it is a smooth muscle innervated by the parasympathetic nervous system. Normally it is contracted. When the bladder muscle contracts to expel urine, this sphincter relaxes and opens.

Lower down, and surrounding the internal sphincter, is the **external sphincter.** This muscle, unlike the internal one, is under voluntary muscular control. Both sphincters act together when there is a urinary reflex (see p. 50).

How the bladder and urethra are situated in the lesser pelvis

By passive supporting elements:

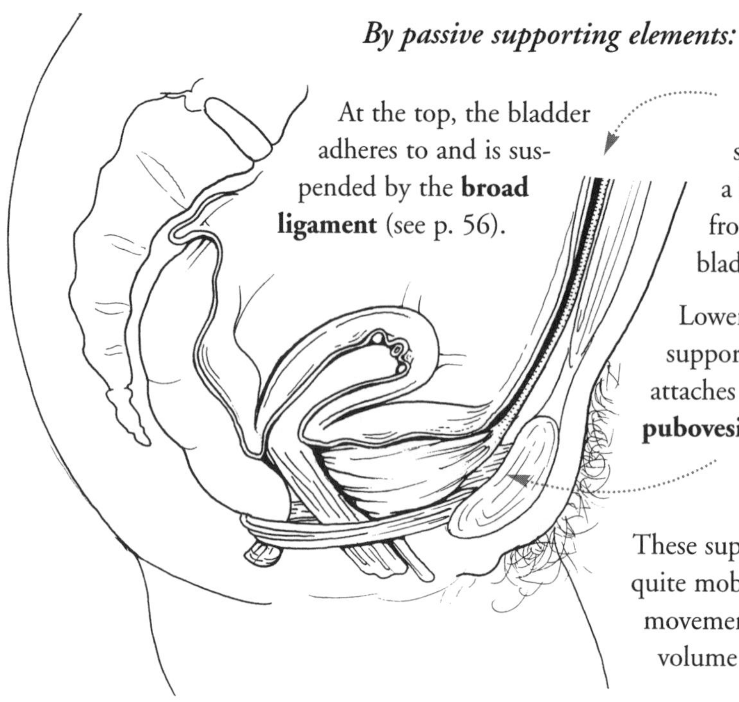

At the top, the bladder adheres to and is suspended by the **broad ligament** (see p. 56).

In front, the bladder is suspended by the **urachus,** a ligament that stretches from the anterior of the bladder to the umbilicus.

Lower down, the bladder is supported by a ligament that attaches it to the pubis, the **pubovesical ligament.**

These supporting elements are quite mobile, which explains the movement that occurs when the volume of the bladder changes.

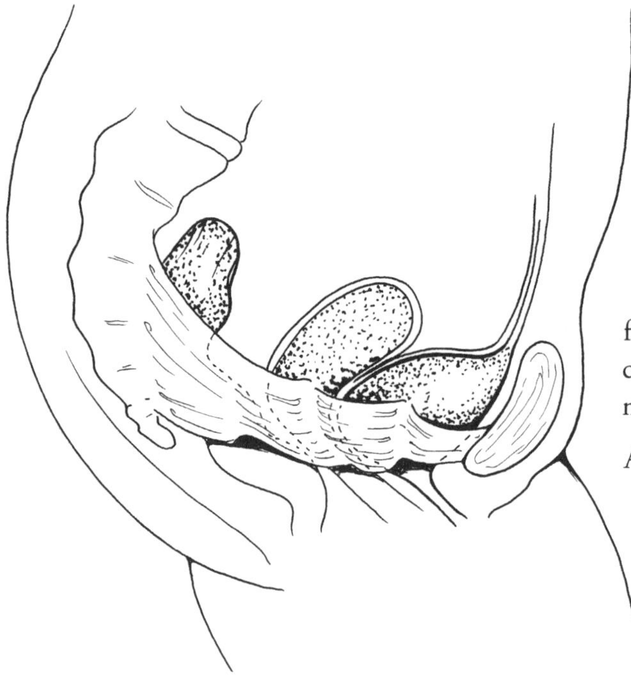

The bladder is strongly fixed. At the back, the base of the bladder and the back of the urethra rest against and adhere to the vagina via a connective tissue, the **vesicovaginal** (or **Halban's) fascia.** Both organs act as if they are stuck together. (This structure is quite fragile and can develop a hernia called **cystocele** [see p. 92] when the muscles of the pelvic floor are weak.)

At the sides, the bladder is bounded by vertical bands of aponeurosis that extend from the sacrum to the pubis (sacrogenital folds).

At the base, the urethra passes through the **perineal membrane,** a fibrous aponeurosis attached to the ischiopubic rami.

By active muscular structures:

There are no muscles directly beneath the bladder and the urethra because the pelvic floor and levator ani form an indentation (or gap) below the organs, the urogenital hiatus (see p. 40).

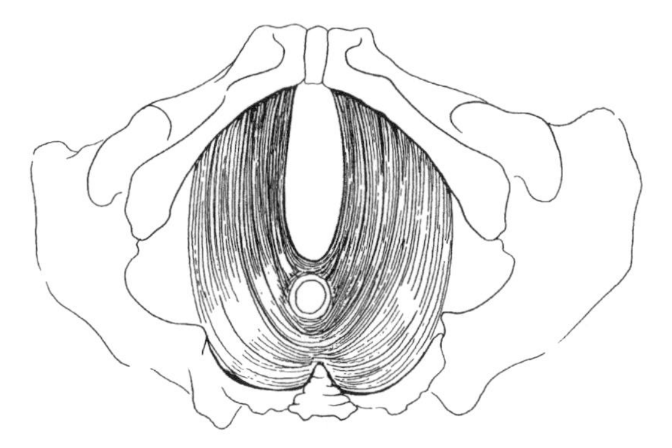

This is the last zone to be stretched during delivery, at the moment of expansion of the anterior perineum (see p. 86).

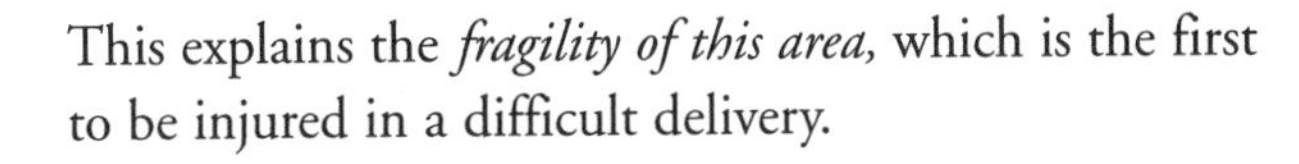

This explains the *fragility of this area,* which is the first to be injured in a difficult delivery.

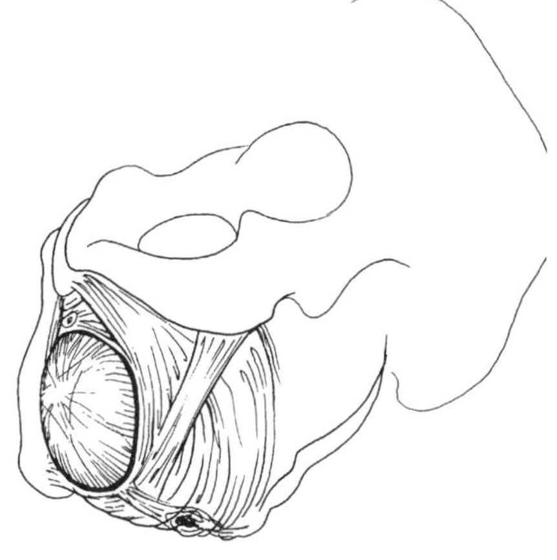

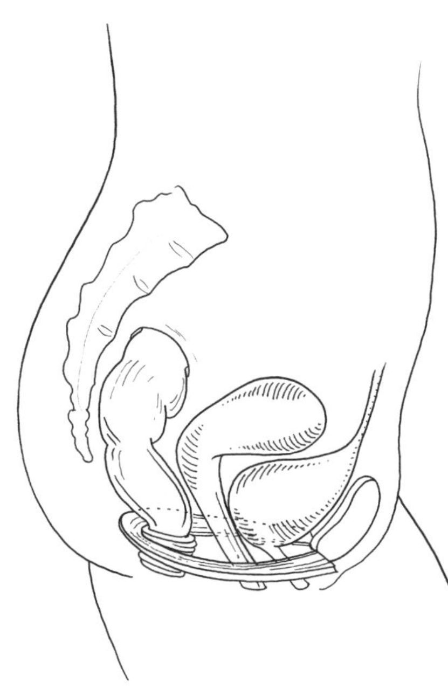

In addition, this is a weak zone since there is no direct support of the pelvic organs from below in this area. The only muscular structures supporting this area are on the sides of the hiatus:

- the deep transverse muscles of the perineum
- the bulbospongiosus muscle
- the puborectalis muscle.

The latter is the most internal section of the levator ani. It is the strongest and most important section to maintain in this region.

Urination

Urination is the act of passing urine.

The urinary reflex mechanism is initiated when the bladder contains approximately 200 milliliters of urine.

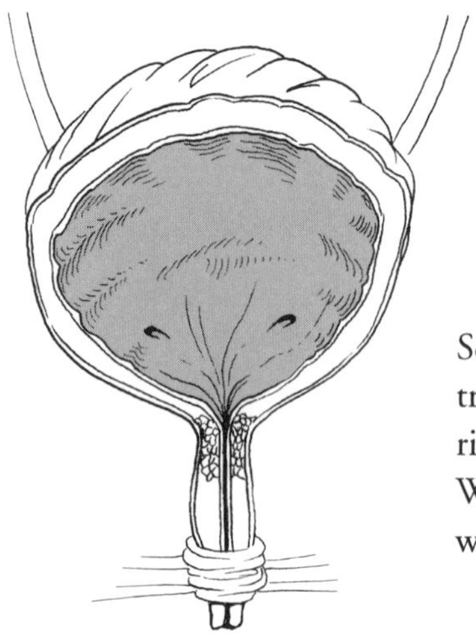

Sensory receptors in the trigone are activated, giving rise to the urge to urinate. We respond in one of two ways:

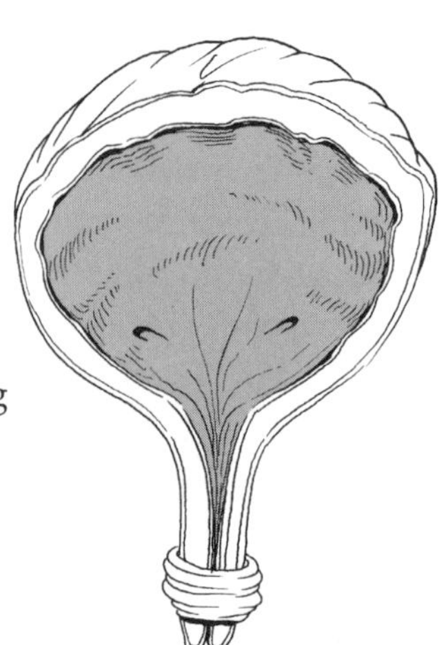

- Urination occurs, as we allow the bladder muscle to contract, and the internal and external sphincters to relax.
- Urination is postponed, as we consciously override the urge to urinate and keep the sphincters contracted. The urge temporarily disappears.

Proper tone of the supporting pelvic floor muscles helps maintain appropriate sphincter function.

The bladder continues to fill until another urge to urinate arises, which can either be responded to or delayed. However, urination becomes unavoidable after successive delays, as the bladder fills even more and the urgency increases.

This reflex system depends on a highly adapted relationship between sensations and the muscular responses of contraction and relaxation.

It is vital to maintain proper functioning of this reflex system, and therefore most important to observe the precautions accompanying the exercise for interrupting urination (see p. 129).

In particular:

- Never stop the same flow more than once, as there is a risk of disturbing the reflex mechanism that signals the need to urinate.
- Only stop near the start of urination, when the pressure is still high.
- Take care to empty the bladder completely when urinating.
- Do not do this at every occasion, just once or twice a day. It is thought that making a habit of interrupting urine flow will upset the reflex mechanism.

These precautions are all repeated in Chapter 8.

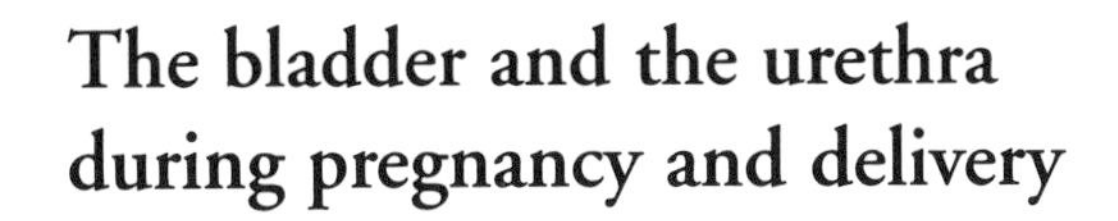

The bladder and the urethra during pregnancy and delivery

During pregnancy, the swollen uterus presses on the bladder. During the three final months, it is not unusual to experience incontinence, as the urethra and the sphincter are stretched and elongated.

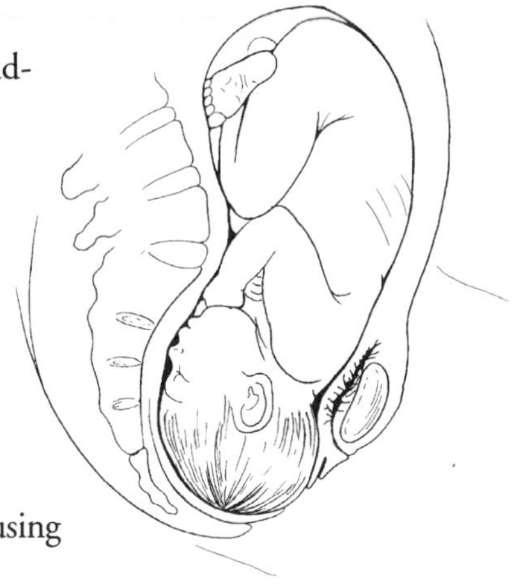

During the delivery, if the bladder is empty, both the bladder and the urethra become compressed during the baby's descent. A full bladder, however, can hamper the baby's descent. It is important to empty the bladder if it is very full, or to pass a small catheter into the bladder if spontaneous urination is not possible.

The elongation of the urethral sphincter is constant: during the phase of expulsion, as the perineal aspect of the vagina dilates, the fibers of its sphincter stretch. As a result, the orientation of the bladder can shift posteriorly, causing future urinary incontinence (see p. 90).

After delivery, two problems can arise:

- The sphincter system can be injured.
- The urge to urinate is no longer felt.

In this case, the bladder can expand upward and prevent the uterus from retracting. Medical attention should then be sought.

Later, during the first two months after delivery, it is common not to be able to entirely stop the flow of urination at will. Incontinence can result from distention of the urinary sphincter during the delivery, or from a ptosis (the bladder occupies a lower place in the pelvis than normal).* Where there are chronic symptoms (see pp. 90 and 91), it is imperative that you see your physician.

During the weeks following this period, *as long as movements involving abdominal hyperpressure are avoided,* all the structures will gradually resume their normal positions. In particular, make sure that you:

- Avoid lifting heavy weights.
- Avoid taking up exercises to strengthen the abdominal muscles too soon, and when you do so, avoid sticking out the lower abdomen and the perineum (see Chapter 8, especially p. 118).

After the delivery, it is suggested that you be examined to determine the state of your perineum, and review these precautions.

---

*This occurs as a result of the bladder falling out of the chamber it usually occupies. Here the pressure interplay between the bladder and urethra has become pathologically reversed: when there is too much pressure on the bladder, it is pushed into the much smaller space usually occupied by the urethra.

The uterus

This is the organ of gestation. It is a hollow muscular organ, triangular in shape, and its extremely vascular internal mucous membrane favors the implantation and development of the fertilized egg.

The uterus is an extensible organ of exceptional strength. Of all the body organs, the uterus is the one that is most able to enlarge itself, which it does during pregnancy (and particularly in multiple pregnancies). It is also capable of considerable and prolonged exertion during the expulsion of the fetus. When a woman is not pregnant, her uterus occupies a relatively small space in the pelvic cavity.

Three parts of the uterus are noteworthy:

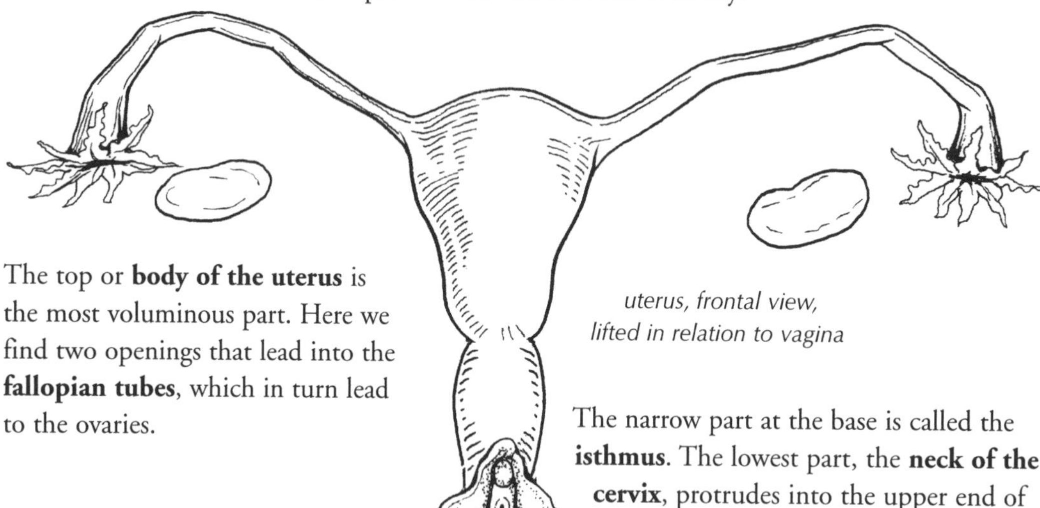

uterus, frontal view, lifted in relation to vagina

The top or **body of the uterus** is the most voluminous part. Here we find two openings that lead into the **fallopian tubes**, which in turn lead to the ovaries.

The narrow part at the base is called the **isthmus**. The lowest part, the **neck of the cervix**, protrudes into the upper end of the vagina.

The mucous membrane lining the uterus is called the **endometrium** and is composed of numerous layers of highly specialized muscular fibers.

The endometrium changes with each ovarian cycle. It thickens at the beginning of the cycle to allow for the embedding of a fertilized ovum. However, if no pregnancy ensues, the tissue is shed during menstruation.

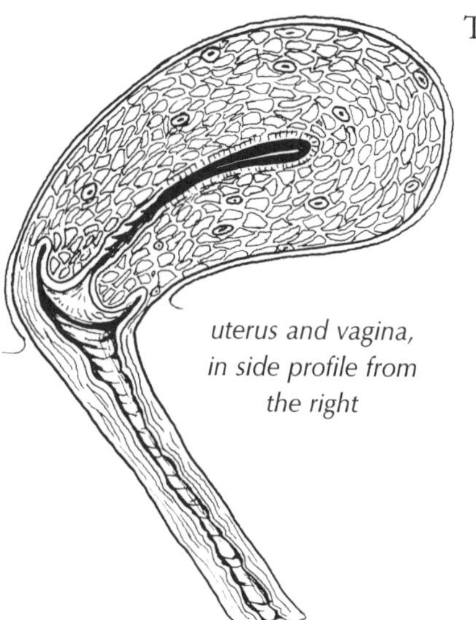

uterus and vagina, in side profile from the right

The uterus is situated in the center of the pelvic cavity, between the bladder in front and the rectum behind.

In profile, we see the forward tilt of the uterus, called anteversion; its slight forward curvature is called anteflexion.

The vagina

This is the organ of sexual intercourse. It is cylindrical in shape (about eight centimeters long) and is situated between the uterus and the vulva. It is slightly concave toward the front, and obliquely inclined 70° toward the back relative to the horizontal.

At the top, the vagina is a little enlarged and attached to the neck of the cervix, which protrudes into it, forming a groove around its circumference (deeper at the back). At its base, the vagina terminates at the vulva. (The constrictor muscles of the vulva close the vaginal orifice.) The anterior and posterior walls of the vagina are virtually touching and are lined with a mucous membrane, forming numerous elastic folds.

The mucous membrane is lined by two layers of muscle:

- a superficial layer with longitudinal fibers
- a deep layer with circular fibers.

These muscular fibers are more developed at the base toward the vaginal opening.

During sexual intercourse, the vaginal mucous membrane stretches open and releases secretions to allow the penis to enter.

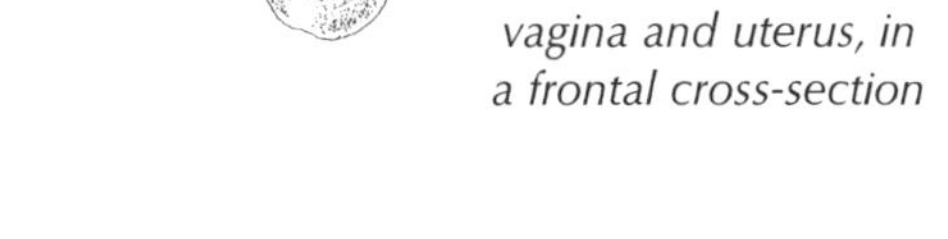

vagina and uterus, in a frontal cross-section

The vagina is located between the bladder and the urethra (in front) and the rectum (behind).

During pregnancy, to facilitate the baby's passage, the mucous membrane becomes much more flexible and elastic.

On the day of the delivery, the tissues stretch out like the pleated folds of an accordion. Tearing of the vagina is thus infrequent or superficial (except when the tissues are in poor condition, as with chronic yeast infections).

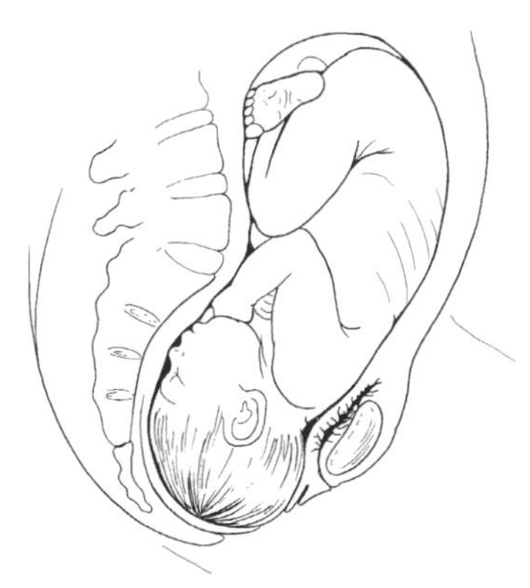

How the uterus and vagina are supported in the lesser pelvis

By their position:

The uterus rests upon and is supported by the bladder, particularly when it is empty, and by the vagina, which acts as a pillar of support. The vagina is held in place from behind by the rectum.

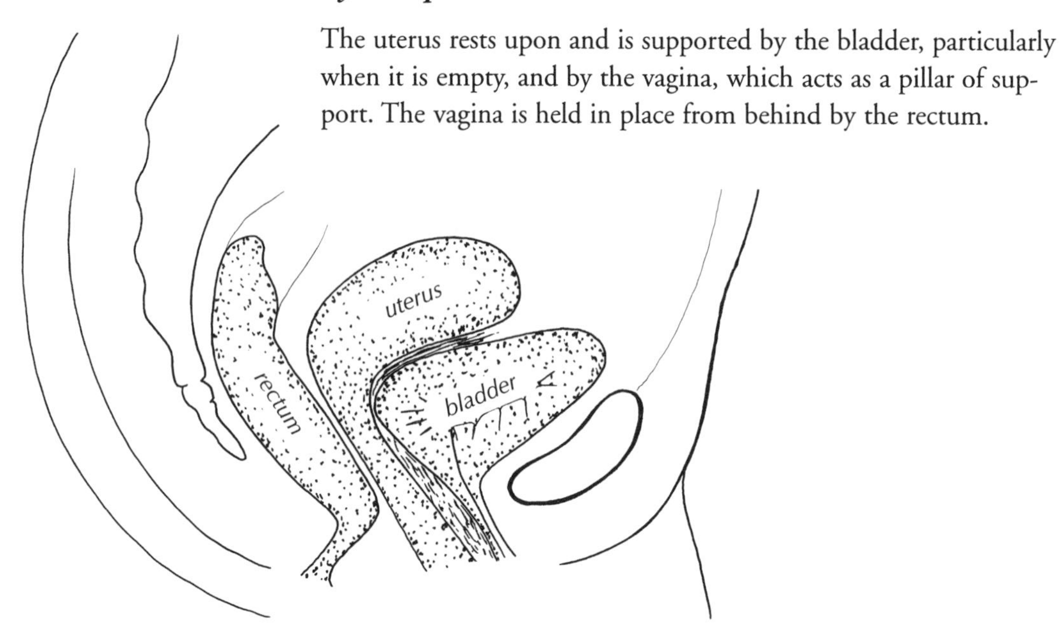

By adhering surfaces:

The posterior underside of the uterus adheres to the bladder through a fascial surface called **rectovesical** (or **Denonvilliers'**) **fascia.** The vagina adheres to the lower part of the bladder (the trigone region) and to the ureter by a common fascial surface called the **vesicovaginal** (or **Halban's**) **fascia.**

By supporting surfaces:

The vagina lies on the perineal membrane, a fibrous layer beneath the deep transverse muscle of the perineum.

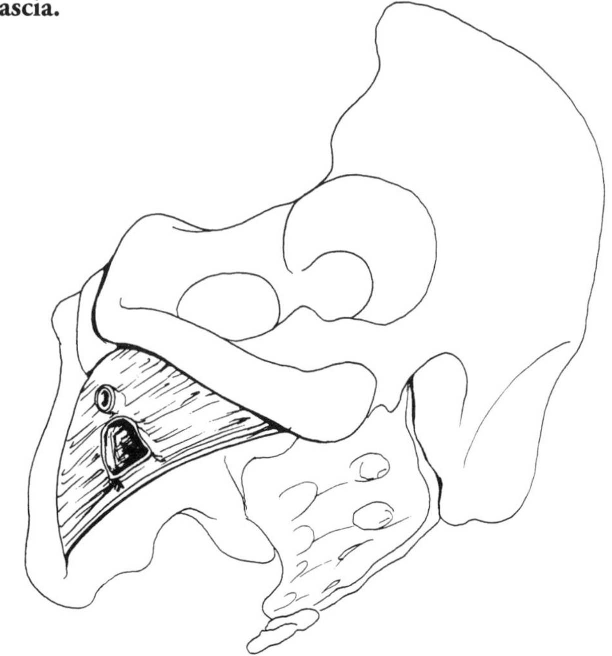

pelvis, seen from below and left

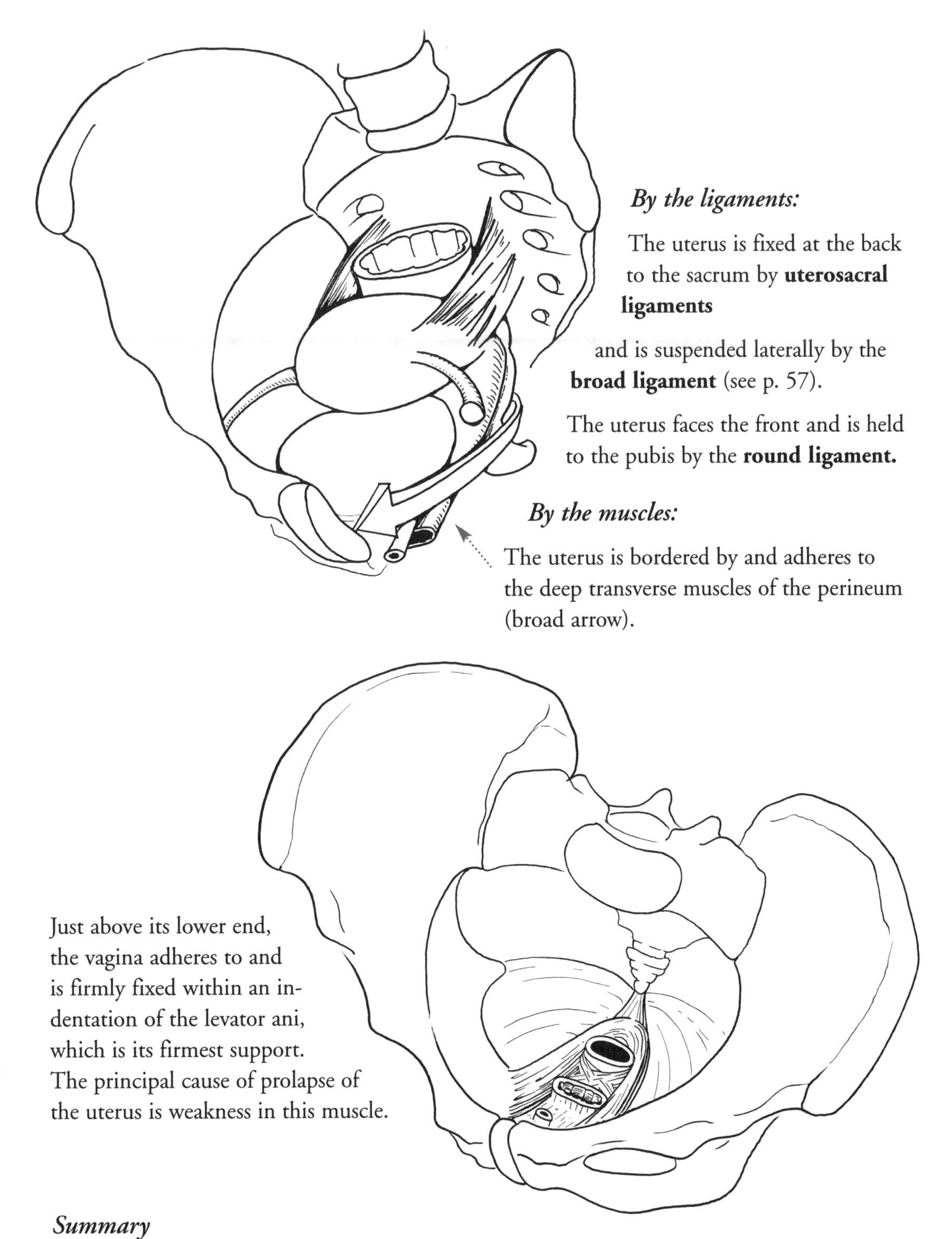

By the ligaments:

The uterus is fixed at the back to the sacrum by **uterosacral ligaments**

and is suspended laterally by the **broad ligament** (see p. 57).

The uterus faces the front and is held to the pubis by the **round ligament.**

By the muscles:

The uterus is bordered by and adheres to the deep transverse muscles of the perineum (broad arrow).

Just above its lower end, the vagina adheres to and is firmly fixed within an indentation of the levator ani, which is its firmest support. The principal cause of prolapse of the uterus is weakness in this muscle.

Summary

The top half (or fundus) of the uterus is quite mobile and its position depends on the degree of fullness of the bladder (in front) or of the rectum (behind). The lower end of the uterus (neck of the cervix) is much more fixed. Lower down in the pelvic cavity the vagina is firmly fixed, and its stability creates a pillar of support for the uterus.

The broad ligament

The abdominal peritoneum covers the pelvic organs and forms deep pouches in front of and behind the uterus:

- the **rectouterine pouch** (pouch of Douglas) at the back
- the **vesicouterine pouch** in the front.

These anterior and posterior folds lie over the uterus, and adhere to each other on the sides. Thus, the uterus is entirely enveloped by the peritoneum.

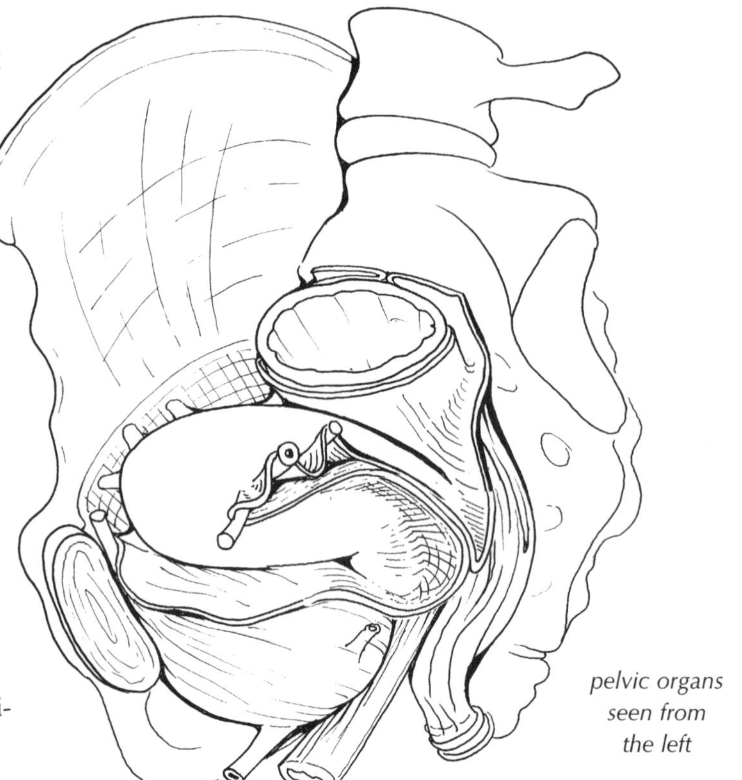

pelvic organs seen from the left

The two adhering layers spread out over the sides and form an ample double partition, called the **broad ligament,** which is attached to the pelvic cavity walls.

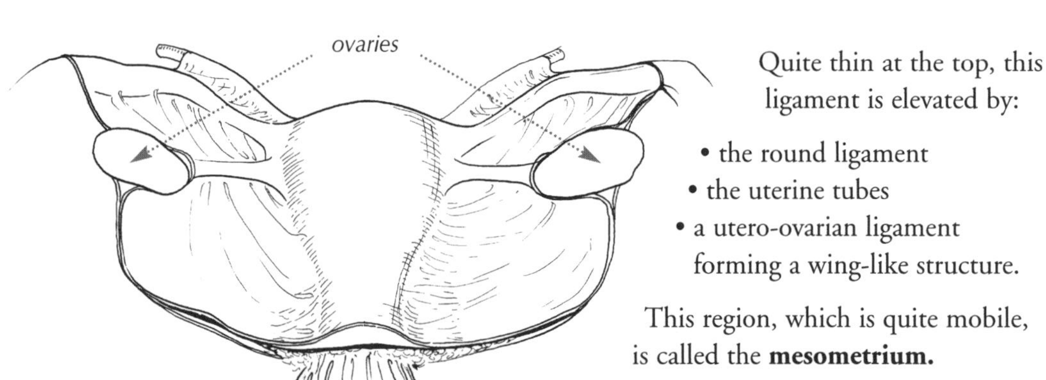

uterus seen vertically from behind to show the spread-out broad ligament

Quite thin at the top, this ligament is elevated by:

- the round ligament
- the uterine tubes
- a utero-ovarian ligament forming a wing-like structure.

This region, which is quite mobile, is called the **mesometrium.**

At the level of the neck of the cervix, the broad ligament is thickened by a dense fibrous strata situated between the two layers. This, unlike other structures in this area, is a fairly immobile region, and it serves to solidly fix the base of the uterus to the edges of the pelvic cavity. This thickened zone is called the **parametrium.** It is traversed by the ureters, blood vessels, and nerves.

The uterus during pregnancy

The uterus begins thickening at the onset of pregnancy, i.e., its muscular fibers are transformed and increase in number. Then the uterus stretches progressively, adapting to the size of the growing fetus.

By week 12, the top of the fetus/uterus reaches a position high in the pelvis. By week 24, it reaches the mid-abdomen, below the navel. By week 36, it reaches the base of the ribs and diaphragm. By week 40, it is much larger, and it descends a little way into the pelvis. It is now said that the fetus is "engaged."

Note: The use of the word *engaged* here at the end of pregnancy is not identical to its use during delivery, where it signifies the beginning of the baby's presentation in the pelvic cavity (see p. 21).

The ligaments holding up the uterus, particularly the uterosacral and round ligaments, adapt to this change. They do this by stretching considerably and by changing their orientation.

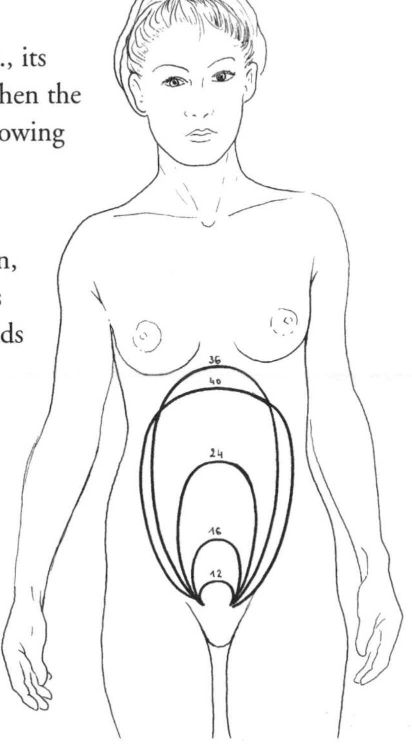

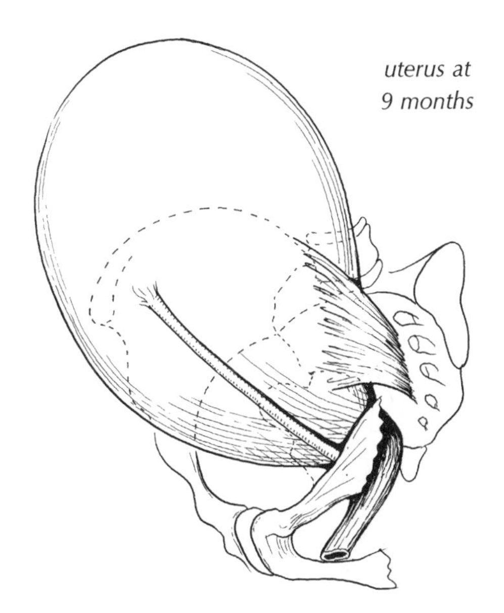

uterus at 9 months

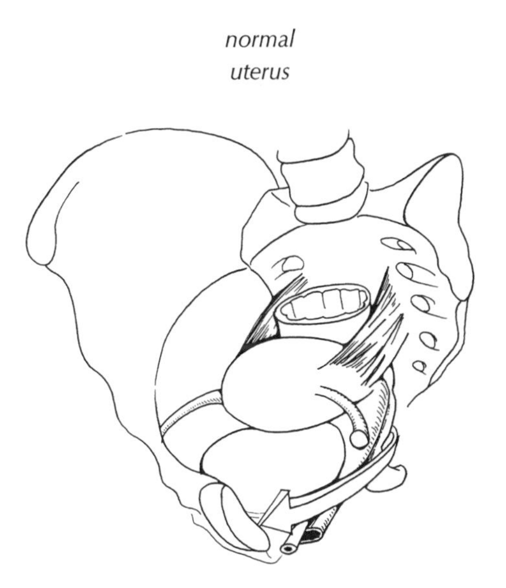

normal uterus

On the day of delivery, contractions of the uterus become stronger, more regular, and more frequent. Their purpose is to dilate the neck of the cervix and expel the baby.

After delivery, the uterus returns to its original size and position in the pelvic cavity within a few hours. Now is the best time to practice the postures that will promote restoration to its normal position (see p. 145).

The rectum

The rectum, also called the rectal ampulla, is located at the end of the large intestine, immediately above the **anus** (terminal orifice). It is situated right at the back of the pelvic cavity, behind the uterus and the vagina.

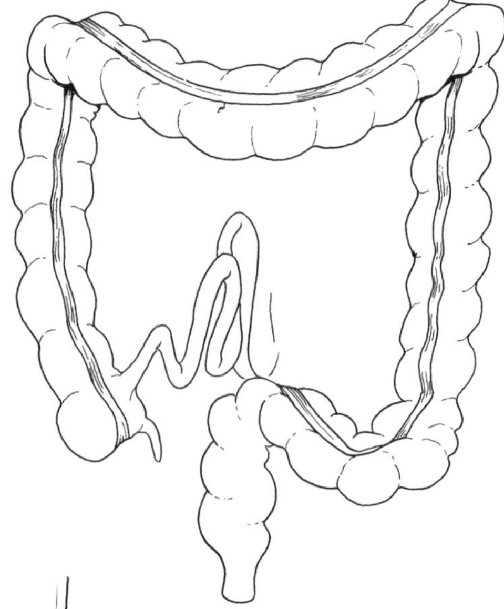

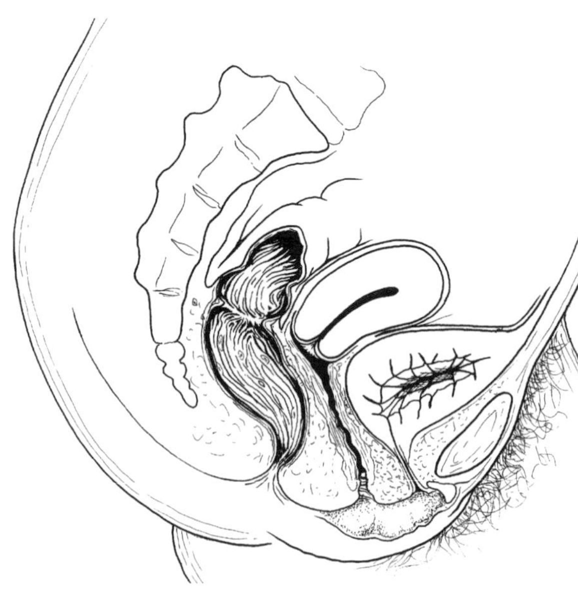

It originates on a level half-way up the sacrum (S-3). In a profile view, you can see that the rectum follows the shape of the sacrum, i.e., it has a curved shape that is concave at the front. Below, having gone through the pelvic floor, it gets thinner and changes its direction, lying obliquely backward and downward to form the **anal canal.**

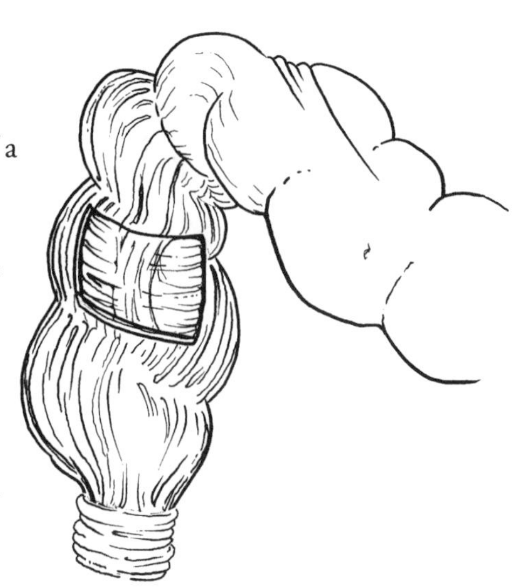

The deeper surfaces of the rectum are made up of a **mucous membrane** that forms longitudinal folds capable of stretching out when the rectum fills. There are also transverse folds, which segment the rectum into valve-like structures.

This mucous membrane is lined with two layers of muscle, the longitudinal muscles and the circular muscles. When these muscles contract, the contents of the rectum are passed out of the body.

The anus

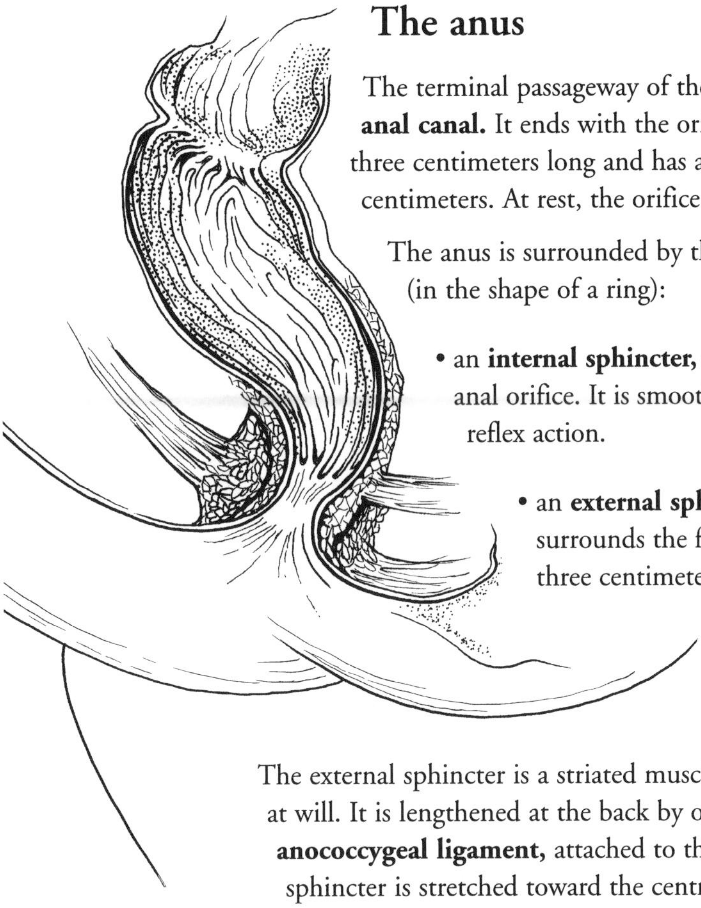

The terminal passageway of the digestive tube is called the **anal canal.** It ends with the orifice called the **anus,** which is three centimeters long and has a diameter of two to three centimeters. At rest, the orifice is closed.

The anus is surrounded by the following sphincter muscles (in the shape of a ring):

- an **internal sphincter,** which directly surrounds the anal orifice. It is smooth visceral muscle that has a reflex action.
- an **external sphincter,** which is bigger and surrounds the first sphincter (approximately three centimeters in length).

The external sphincter is a striated muscle that can contract and relax at will. It is lengthened at the back by overlapping fibers called the **anococcygeal ligament,** attached to the coccyx. In front, the external sphincter is stretched toward the central tendon of the perineum.

Finally, the anus goes through the layer of levator ani muscle, and the external sphincter adheres to its fibers.

This crossover area is called the **anal angle.**

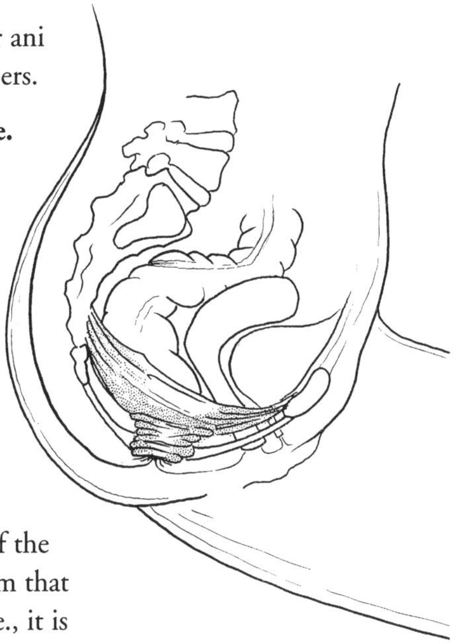

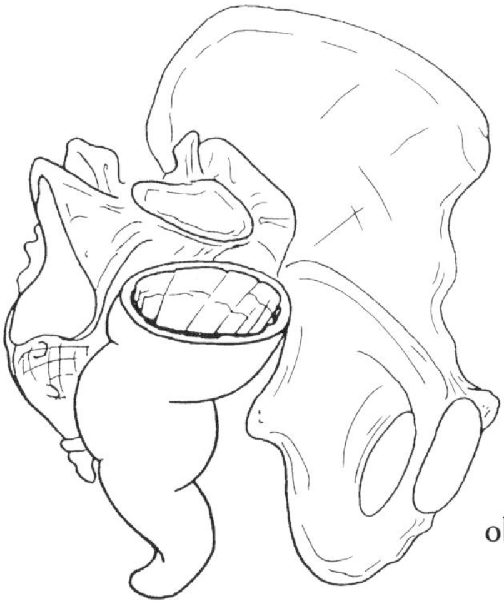

From this point, the direction of the anus differs from that of the rectum, i.e., it is oblique toward the back.

How the rectum and anus are supported in the pelvis

By passive supporting structures:

The top of the rectum, which is an extension of the large intestine, is covered by the peritoneum, to which it adheres. The peritoneal folds in this area are the:

- retrorectal fold at the back
- laterorectal fold at the sides
- rectouterine pouch (or pouch of Douglas) at the front.

Further down, the rectum is bordered along its sides by the sacrogenital folds.

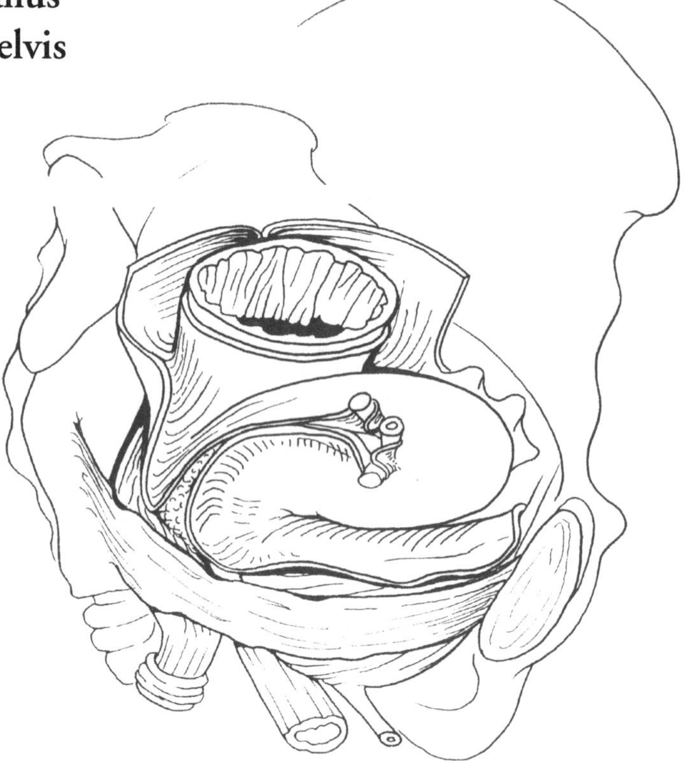

By active muscular structures:

The most external fascia of the levator ani borders and supports the rectum. The fascia, however, does not adhere to it, thus permitting variations in its volume.

The anal canal is more fixed in position. Its fibers merge with those of the puborectalis part of the levator ani.

Lower down, the external sphincter is attached:

- at the back to the coccyx by the anococcygeal ligament, which merges its upper fibers into those of the levator ani
- in front to the central tendon of the perineum (see p. 42).

Because of these attachments, this region of the anal canal and the anus do not collapse, even when there is a prolapse of the rectum.

Defecation

Like urination, defecation (the act of emptying the bowels) is a combination of voluntary and involuntary actions.

When the rectum is filled, sensitive nerve receptors are activated and the urge to defecate is felt. A reflex response occurs: the muscular walls of the rectum contract and the internal sphincter relaxes. Waste matter moves into the lowest part of the rectum to be evacuated. At this point, one of two situations may occur:

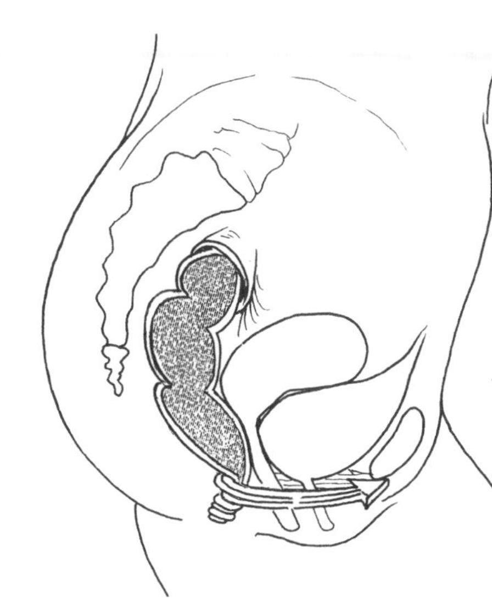

Evacuation is not immediately possible (fecal continence). This is the result of contraction by one of two sets of voluntary muscles, either the striated sphincter of the anus or the levator ani (especially the puborectalis muscle). The contraction of the levator acts like a girth strap and accentuates the anal angle, which pulls the anus toward the front and flattens out the opening against itself. Most importantly, the urge to evacuate disappears. It will reappear later when the rectum has filled more.

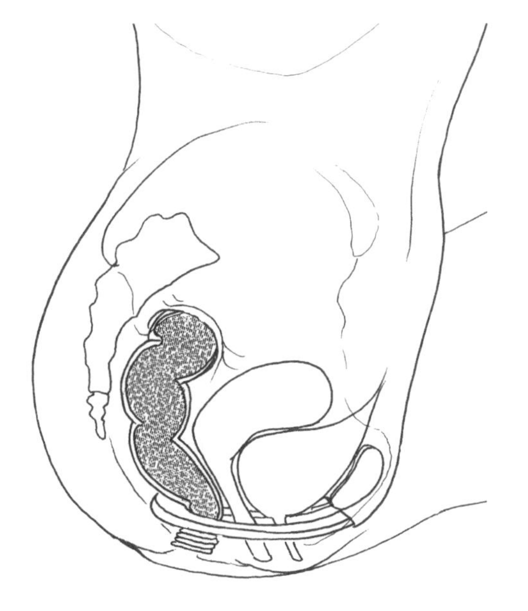

Evacuation is immediately possible. The striated sphincter and the puborectalis bundle relax, thereby easing the anal angle. At this moment the rectum and anus are almost aligned, and the anal orifice, no longer flattened, is able to open.

This reflex system is under the control of the parasympathetic nervous system. Its proper function depends on being well-adjusted to sensations and both voluntary and involuntary responses. It is important to maintain this balance, or to restore it if it has been upset by a particular habit or lifestyle (see exercises on pp. 132-135).

CHAPTER FOUR

The Muscles Bordering the Perineum

When you first try to feel the sensation associated with muscular contraction in the pelvic floor, you may find instead that you are discovering and using the following neighboring muscles:

- deep hip muscles
- adductor muscles
- gluteal muscles
- lower abdominal muscles.

While performing the following exercises, you will often find that these muscles contract at *the same time as the perineum—and maybe even instead of it.*

Why? Quite simply, because they are bigger and are called upon more often in everyday living. It is normal to confuse their contraction with that of the perineum itself.

This is not a problem unless the muscles bordering the perineum prevent an awareness of the actual pelvic floor. For this reason, it will be useful to get to know these muscles and to pinpoint the sites of their contractions. That will allow you to distinguish them easily from those of the perineum. In addition, you will learn how to use the neighboring muscles in different situations, at the same time as you use some or all of the perineal muscles.

Finally, we will look at the diaphragm. Even though this muscle is situated far from the pelvis, it is functionally linked to the perineum.

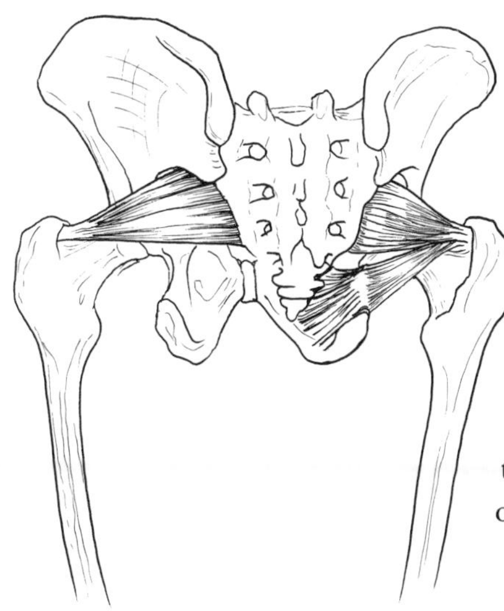

The deep hip muscles

These muscles are attached to the pelvis and extend outward to a protusion at the top of the femur called the **greater trochanter.** They are principally involved in external rotation of the hip.

The **piriformis muscle** is attached to the lower internal surface of the sacrum and runs forward and outward, leaving the pelvis and ending at the top of the femur. It is right next to the rectum, and its contraction is often mistaken for that of the posterior fascia of the levator ani.

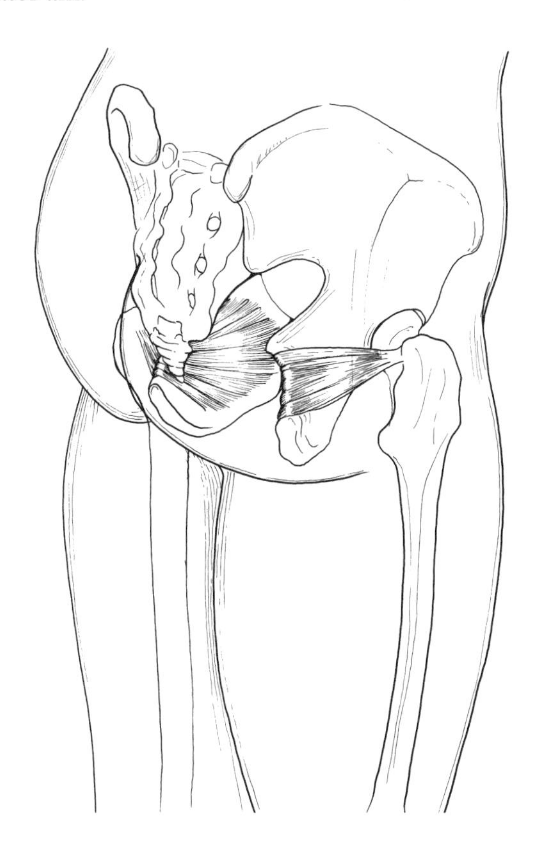

The **obturator internus muscle** is attached within the pelvic cavity, covering the obturator foramen. Thus, it is extremely close to the pelvic floor muscles before it folds over itself and leaves the pelvis to run toward the femur.

To isolate these two muscles and thereby keep them out of play, we will use a cross-legged position (see bottom of p. 67).

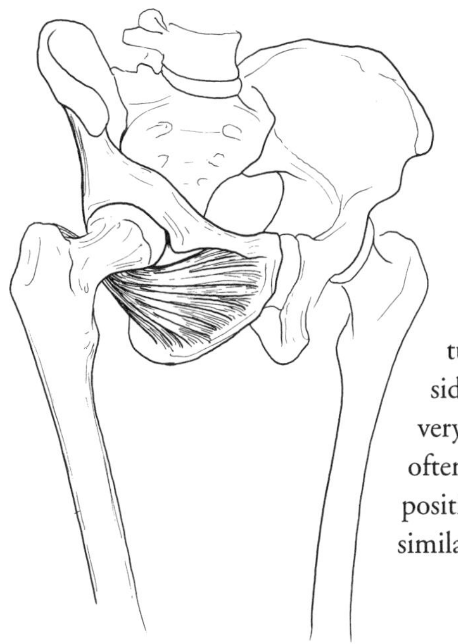

The **obturator externus muscle** also crosses the obturator foramen, but on the opposite surface (external side of the pelvis). Then it runs toward the femur. It is very close to the deep adductors and its contractions are often mistaken for those of the anterior perineum. The positions that will be used to distinguish this muscle are similar to those for the adductor muscles (see p. 67).

The gluteal muscles

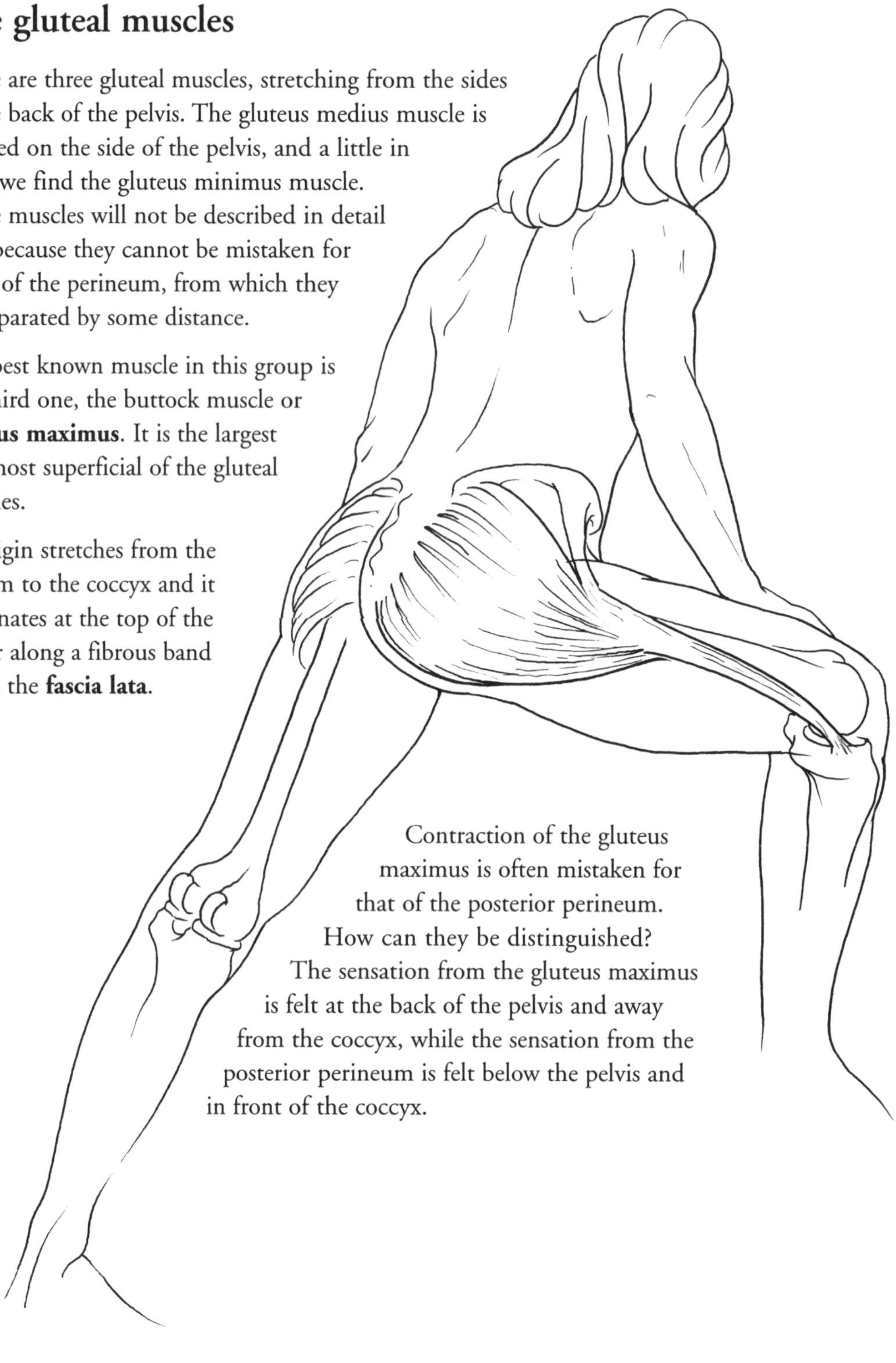

There are three gluteal muscles, stretching from the sides to the back of the pelvis. The gluteus medius muscle is situated on the side of the pelvis, and a little in front we find the gluteus minimus muscle. These muscles will not be described in detail here because they cannot be mistaken for those of the perineum, from which they are separated by some distance.

The best known muscle in this group is the third one, the buttock muscle or **gluteus maximus**. It is the largest and most superficial of the gluteal muscles.

Its origin stretches from the sacrum to the coccyx and it terminates at the top of the femur along a fibrous band called the **fascia lata**.

Contraction of the gluteus maximus is often mistaken for that of the posterior perineum. How can they be distinguished? The sensation from the gluteus maximus is felt at the back of the pelvis and away from the coccyx, while the sensation from the posterior perineum is felt below the pelvis and in front of the coccyx.

How to distinguish between the perineal and the gluteus maximus muscles

The positions described below enable one to distinguish between the perineal and gluteus maximus muscles while exercising the muscles of the posterior perineum—the posterior fascia of the levator ani, the anal sphincters, and the rectal muscles.

To begin with, *take the gluteus maximus muscle out of play* by flexing the thighs. This can be done by either:

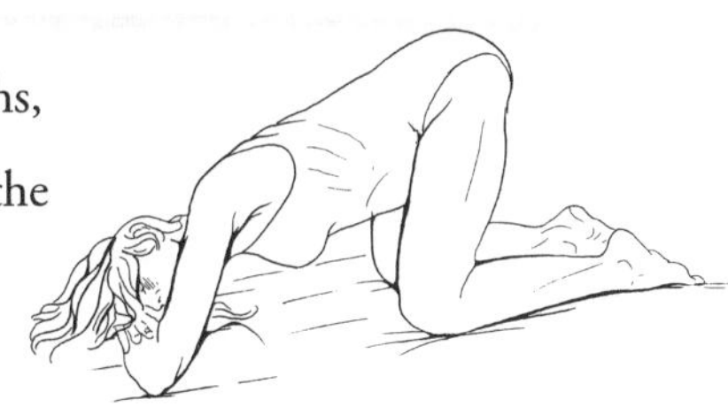

lying on your back and lifting the thighs against the chest,

squatting,

sitting on your thighs,

kneeling on the floor, and extending your upper body forward,

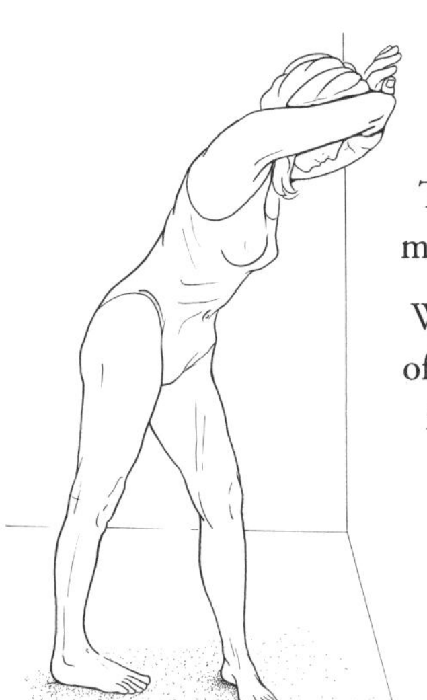

or turning the leg inward (while standing) and crossing one knee over the other (the hips are thereby adducted).

This makes it more difficult to activate the gluteal muscles and easier to identify those of the perineum.

When you have clearly experienced the contraction of the posterior perineal muscles, try exercising them in a position that makes it more difficult to isolate the different sets of muscles, for example:

during hip extension (right),

or by sitting with your legs wide apart.

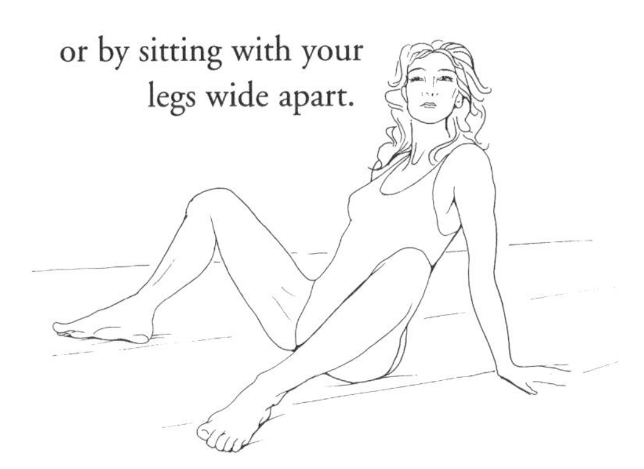

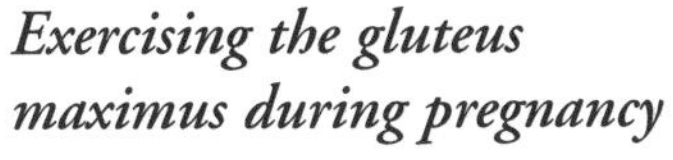

Exercising the gluteus maximus during pregnancy

As a result of the particular hormones released during pregnancy, the pelvic joints are more flexible, sometimes even too flexible (see p. 28). There could be a feeling of instability (e.g., that the pelvis might "break") and of pain. The gluteus maximus muscle covers the sacroiliac joints. For this reason, it can, when it is toned, help "tighten" the pelvis. Exercises to reinforce the muscles are proposed for this purpose (see pp. 122 and 123).

The adductor muscles

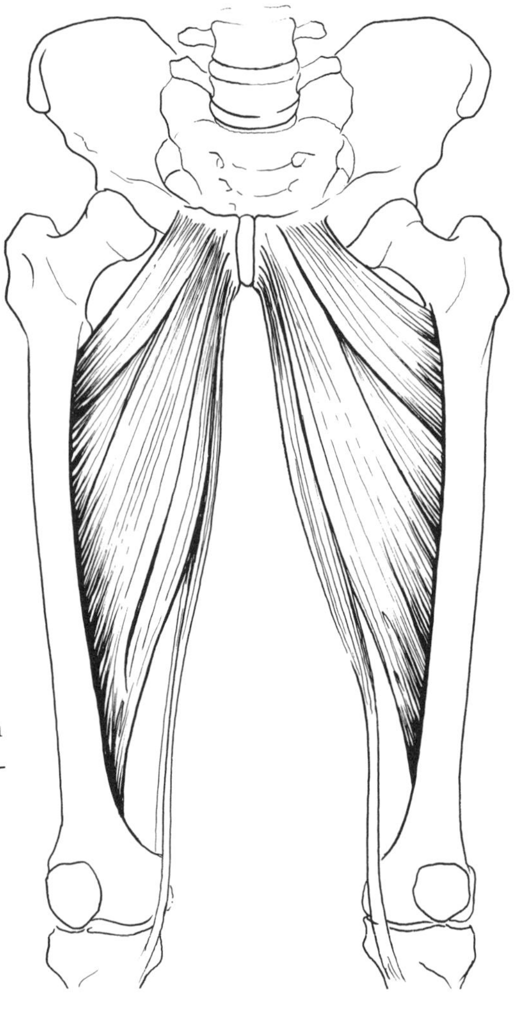

These muscles are found on the inside of the thigh. There are five of them, each one longer than the other, with the outermost muscles covering the innermost muscles.

Three small muscles stretch between the upper part of the pubis and the head of the femur:

- the **pectineus**
- the **adductor minimus**
- the **adductor brevis**.

Then there are two longer ones:

- the **adductor magnus** and
- the **gracilis muscle**, which stretches as far as the knee and is attached to the top of the tibia.

These muscles draw the thighs together. They are close to the pelvis, and thus their contraction can be mistaken for that of the anterior perineal muscles.

However, when the adductor muscles are contracted, the sensations are experienced in the inside of the thighs, not in the lower pelvis.

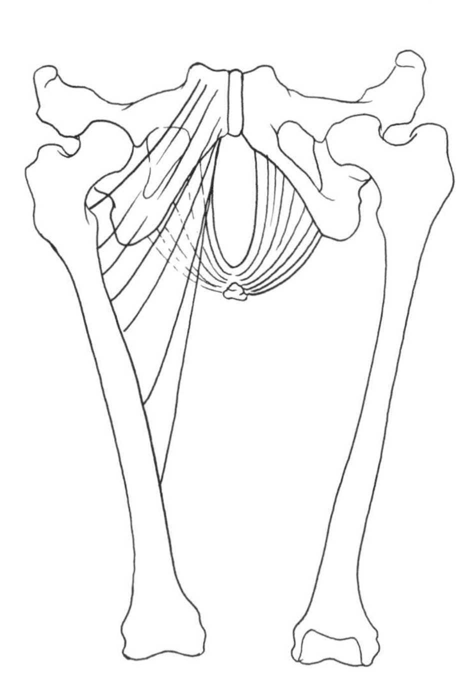

Here, the pelvis is seen from the front, and slightly from below, showing the levator ani muscles (behind the pubis) and the upper adductors (attached to the right leg).

The day of delivery

It is important for the adductor muscles to be supple, allowing the thighs to open easily when sitting, squatting, or lying down. See the exercises for identifying, loosening up, and toning the adductors on p. 124.

How to distinguish between the adductor and anterior perineal muscles

The positions described below allow one to distinguish between the adductor and anterior perineal muscles while exercising the muscles of the anterior perineum, the anterior sections of the levator ani, and the urethral sphincter.

It helps to stretch out the adductors by opening the thighs. This can be done by:

squatting with the knees apart,

standing up and extending one knee to the side, while stepping on a support (this allows you to isolate each side from the other),

or sitting with the thighs wide apart.

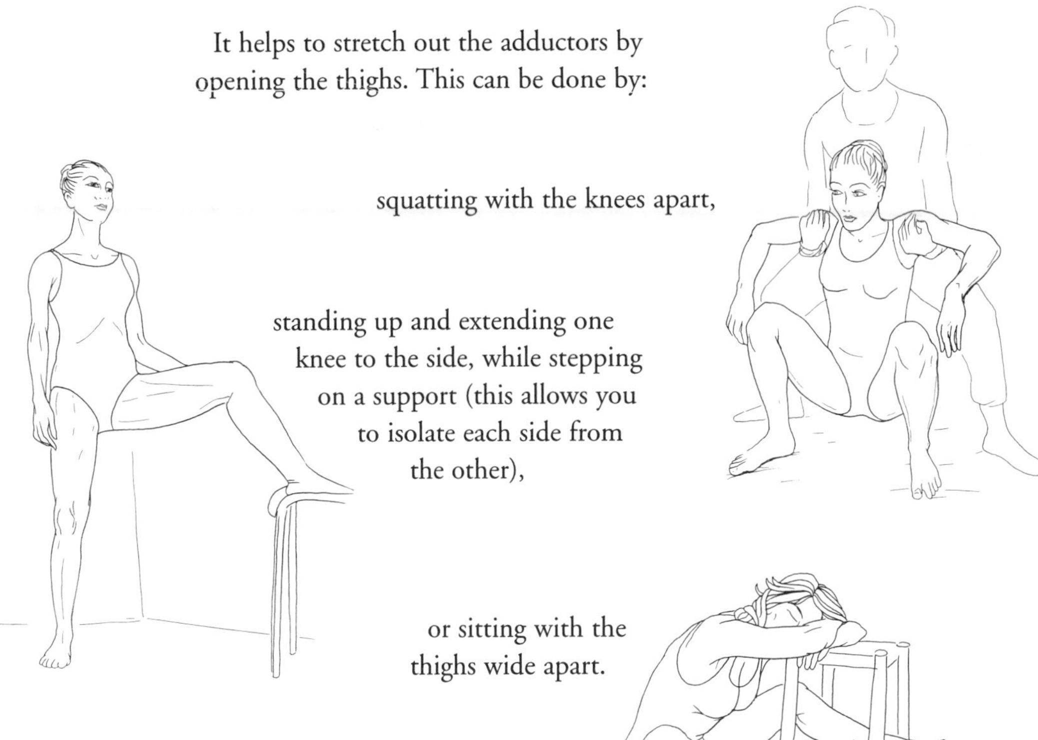

These positions make it more difficult to activate the adductor muscles, thereby making it easier to find the muscles of the perineum.

Avoid positions in which the thighs are close together or the knees are slightly flexed. These positions facilitate the contraction of the adductors, and thus make it harder to appreciate the movement of the perineal muscles.

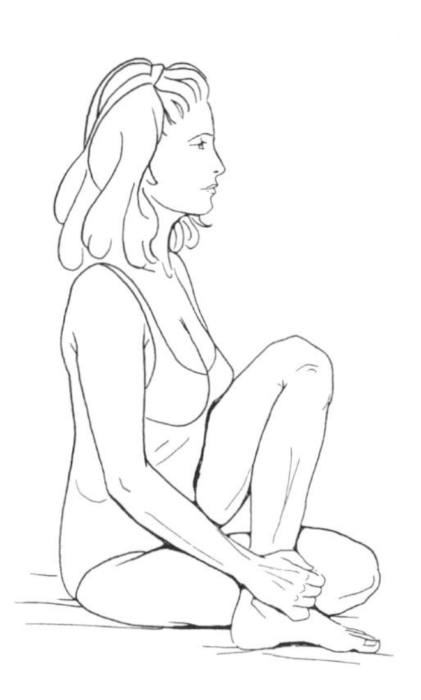

Eventually, once you have clearly felt the differences between the two sets of muscles, you can try contracting the perineal muscles in normal, everyday positions, even though it might be harder to distinguish between them.

The abdominal muscles

These muscles are situated between the ribs and the pelvis. There are two common misconceptions about this region and these muscles:

- The abdomen is *not* limited to the region of the abdominal muscles. Its upper part extends beneath the ribs.
- The abdominal muscles are *not* confined to just the front of the trunk. Rather, most of these muscles are located on the sides, and actually even behind, as illustrated below.

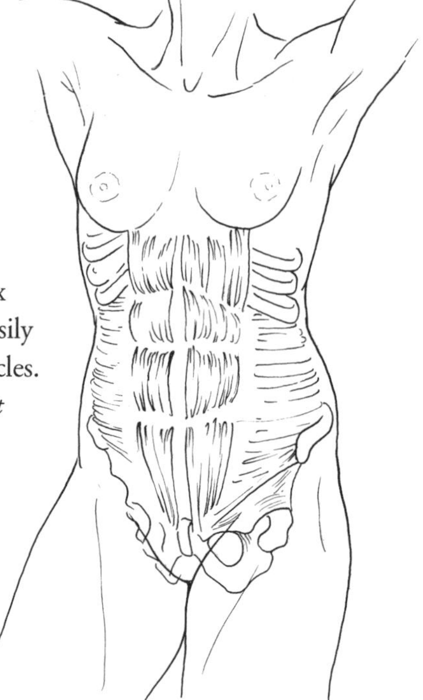

The **rectus abdominis muscle** is found entirely along the front of the body. It stretches from the front of the thorax (sternum) as far as the pubis, and has long fibers that are easily felt. The lower fibers are close to the anterior perineal muscles. Of all the abdominal muscles, *it is these fibers that are most commonly mistaken for those of the perineum.*

The abdominal muscles form three successive layers over the sides of the trunk. They stretch from the sides to the pelvis. They are attached at the back to the lumbar vertebrae and in the front to a wide aponeurosis.

The deepest muscles in this group are the **transverses abdominis muscles.** Their fibers are horizontal. Thus, when they are contracted, they pull the diameter of the abdomen inward, as if tightening a belt. These are the muscles that assist in *exhaling the breath,* particularly deep breaths. You can feel them in the lower rib region when exhaling deeply, or when sneezing or coughing.

The **internal and external oblique muscles** interweave their fibers to stretch across the transverse muscles. The oblique muscles contribute to the squeezing of the abdomen during exhalation. They also mobilize the trunk, enabling the thorax and pelvis to turn or lean against each other.

These muscles stretch a great deal during pregnancy, which makes it vital that they be exercised after the delivery, with certain precautions (see pp. 118-121 and 146). The abdominal muscles serve different roles during delivery (see pp. 72-74).

Reinforcing the abdominal and perineal muscles

When the abdominal muscles contract together, the result is a pulling in of the waist (or the abdomen). Since the abdomen as such is incompressible (it can be compared to a volume of liquid), the effect of squeezing it in at the waist necessarily displaces it elsewhere, i.e., either:

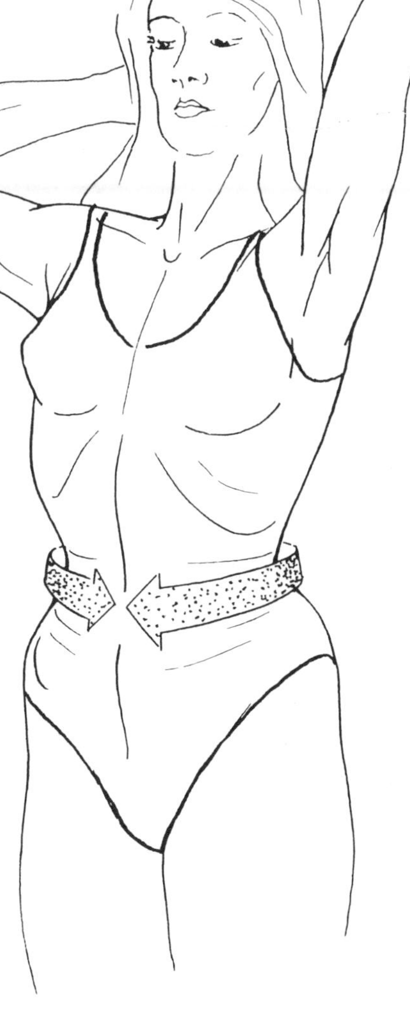

- *upward,* in which case the abdomen presses against the thorax during a long exhalation, to help the lungs empty themselves
- *downward,* in which case the abdomen presses on the perineum during acts of expulsion
- *both upward and downward,* which occurs most commonly.

Excessive pressure can be put on the perineum while exercising the abdominal muscles, especially if the waist is pulled in, in an exaggerated manner, to make an "hourglass" figure, and the lower abdomen (i.e., the muscles of the lower abdomen and pelvic floor) lacks the proper tone.

Such pressure sometimes creates difficulties for the perineum, particularly when it has been weakened by:

- pregnancy
- the presence of lesions (tears or episiotomy) after delivery
- loss of tonicity
- the presence of a prolapse.

In such cases, exercises to reinforce the abdominal muscles would have a negative effect on the perineum if they:

- create a downward pressure
- distend the lower abdomen or perineum.

Exercises for the abdominal muscles should be preceded by contraction of the muscles of the pelvic floor, to stabilize it.

Exercises for these muscles are described on pp. 118-121, and in the section on pregnancy, pp. 140-146.

The diaphragm

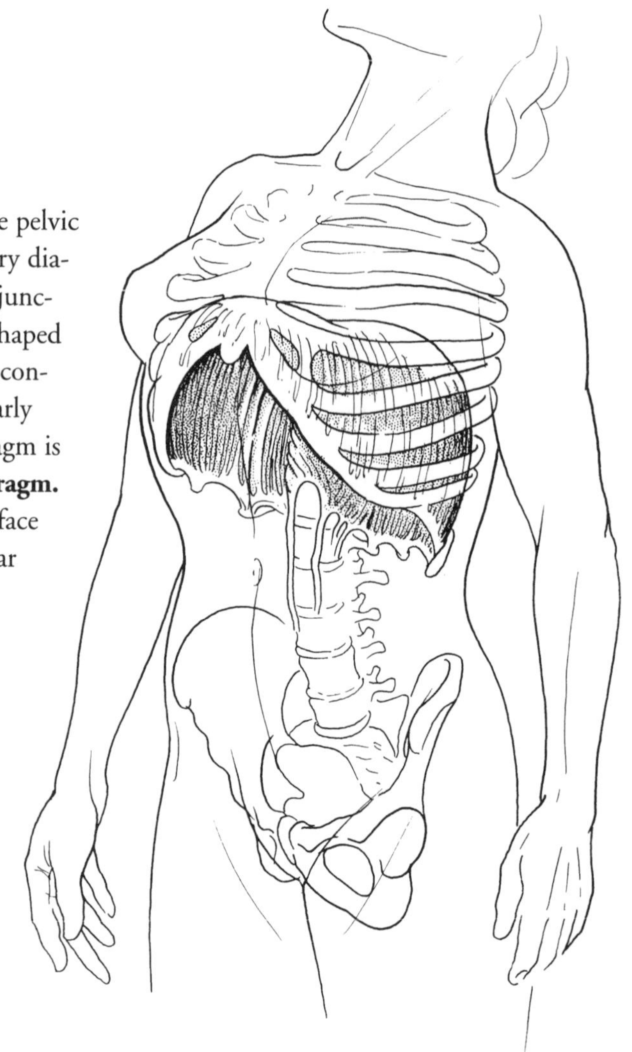

The pelvic floor is sometimes called the pelvic diaphragm, in contrast to the respiratory diaphragm, which is located above at the junction of the abdomen and the thorax. Shaped like a dome, the top of the diaphragm contains a noncontractile fibrous zone, pearly white in color. This part of the diaphragm is called the **central tendon of the diaphragm.** Fibers radiate outward to the inner surface of the thorax, sternum, ribs, and lumbar vertebra.

This is the *major muscle used during inhalation.*

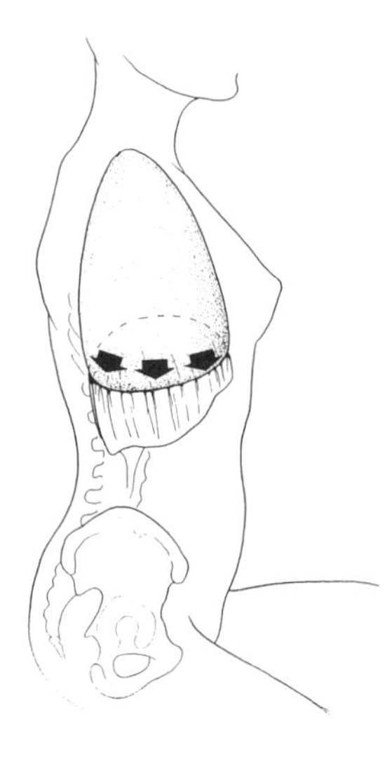

Its actions are complex. Here is a simplified explanation:

When the muscular fibers along its rim contract, the central tendon descends. This expands the lungs toward their base. Thus stretched, the lungs fill up with air, i.e., they inhale.

Conversely, during exhalation, the opposite occurs. The diaphragm moves upward, accompanying the lungs as they return to their original size.

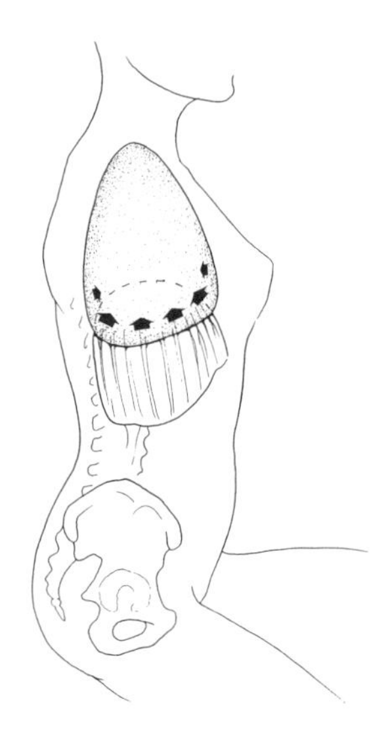

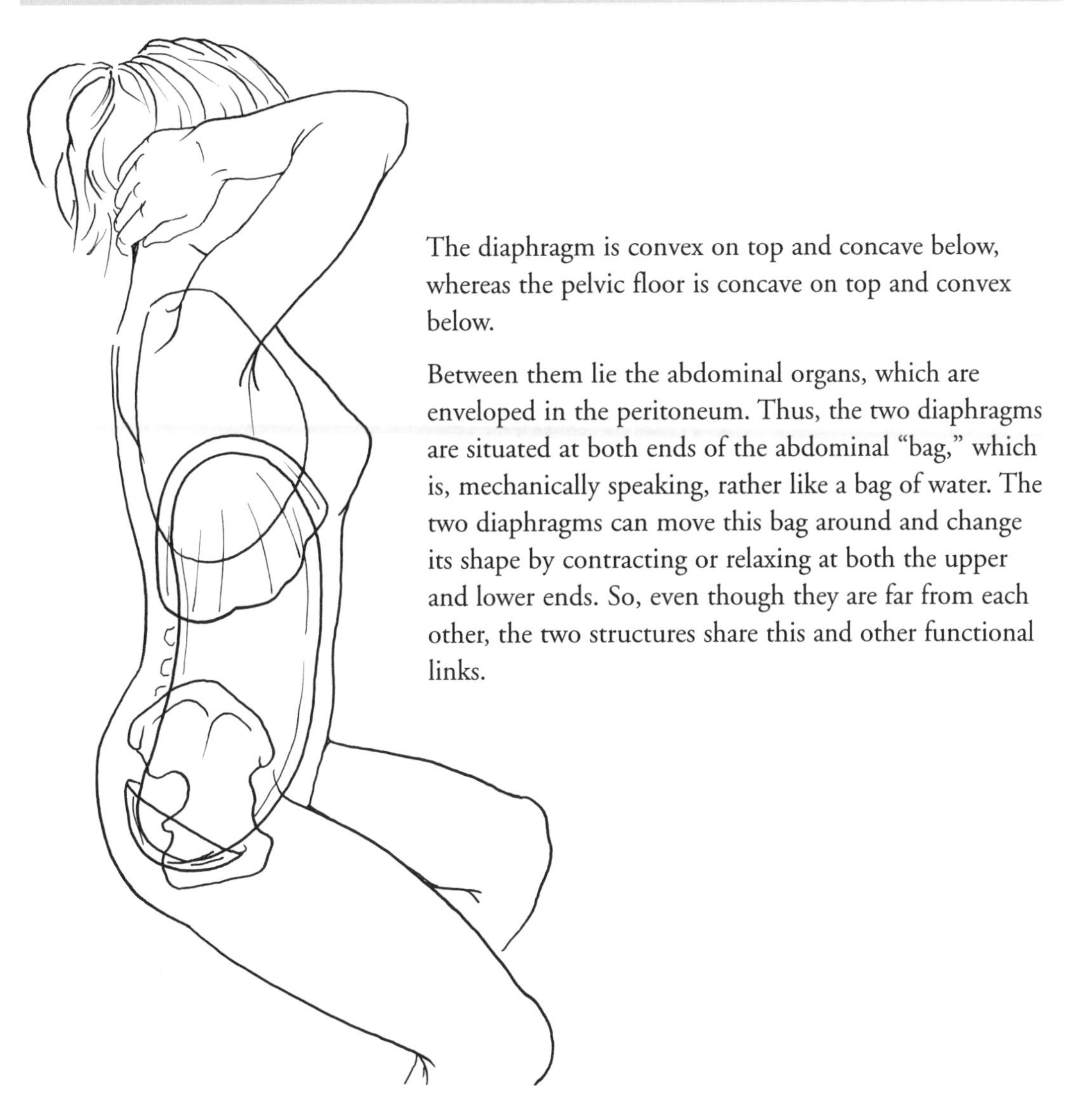

The diaphragm is convex on top and concave below, whereas the pelvic floor is concave on top and convex below.

Between them lie the abdominal organs, which are enveloped in the peritoneum. Thus, the two diaphragms are situated at both ends of the abdominal "bag," which is, mechanically speaking, rather like a bag of water. The two diaphragms can move this bag around and change its shape by contracting or relaxing at both the upper and lower ends. So, even though they are far from each other, the two structures share this and other functional links.

The diaphragm during expulsion

The movements of the diaphragm are associated with other functions besides breathing, such as digestion, circulation, coughing, and speaking. In particular, the diaphragm's movements join those of other muscles in the following acts of expulsion:

- *defecation*
- *urination* (if need be)
- in the final phase of *delivery,* where it plays a different role.

The second or final stage of delivery is precisely called **expulsion** (see p. 85). This process provokes a very different sensation in the mother from that experienced during the dilation of the cervix: an uncontrollable desire to *push,* followed by strong contractions of the uterine muscles. This is the **expulsive reflex,** which is provoked by the pressure of the fetus upon the perineum.

However, if the dilatation is completed and the mother is encouraged to push prematurely, the reflex will not occur. Similarly, the use of an epidural injection will obliterate the natural sensations and the reflex will be absent.

Let us start by identifying the forces at work during the second stage that contribute to the act of delivery.

The **diaphragm,** situated above, can contract downward and push somewhat like a piston.

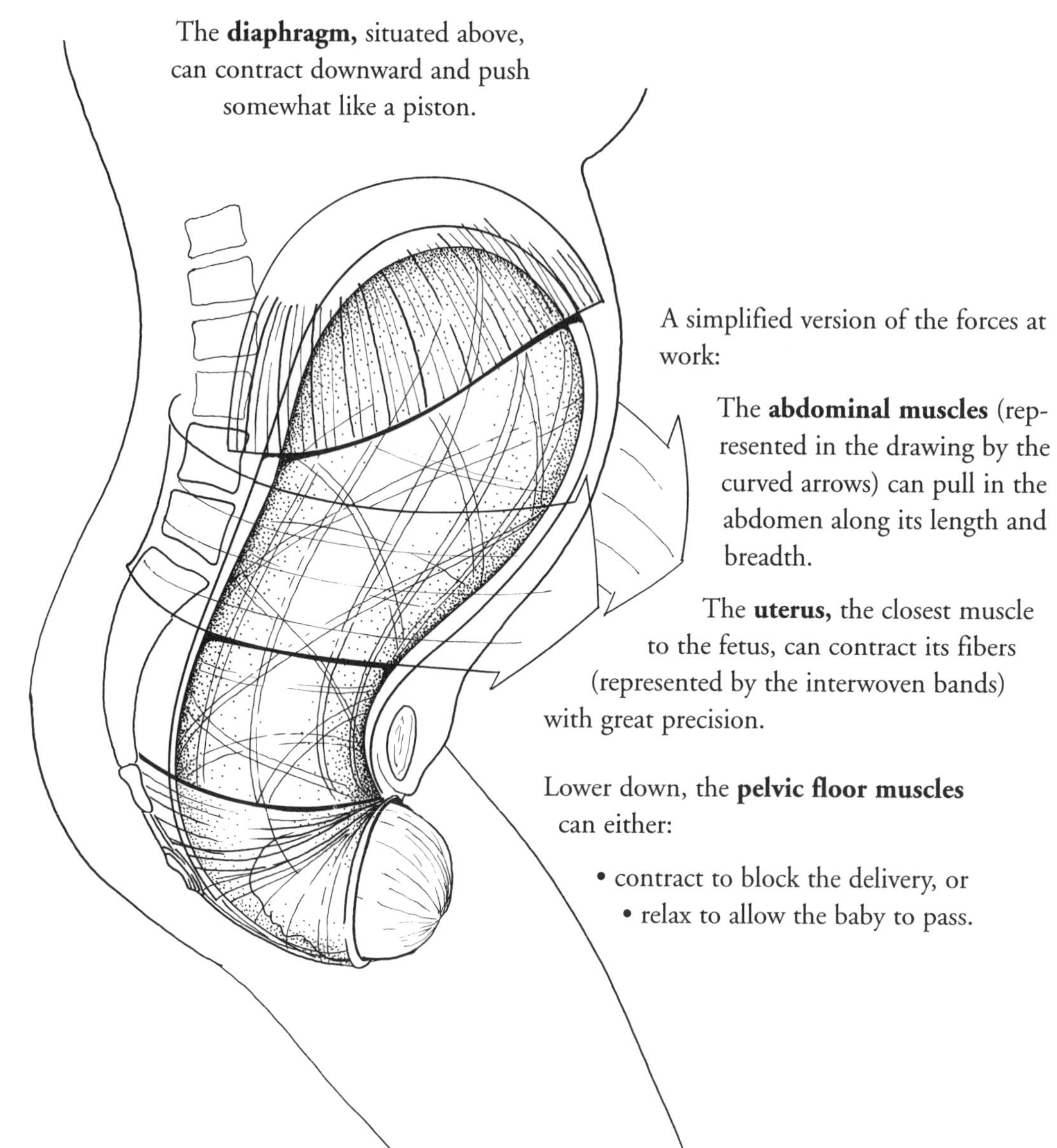

A simplified version of the forces at work:

The **abdominal muscles** (represented in the drawing by the curved arrows) can pull in the abdomen along its length and breadth.

The **uterus,** the closest muscle to the fetus, can contract its fibers (represented by the interwoven bands) with great precision.

Lower down, the **pelvic floor muscles** can either:

- contract to block the delivery, or
- relax to allow the baby to pass.

Finally, it is important to remember that, depending on the position assumed during delivery, the **weight factor** (or gravity) has a role to play in the act of expulsion. As shown above, the delivery is taking place in an upright position. The weight factor will enable the baby to move toward and out of the perineum. But if you turn the page around so that the trunk is in a horizontal position, you can readily see that the weight factor would no longer be of any help, and could even hinder the second stage of expulsion.

How the diaphragm acts when pushing with a blocked inhalation

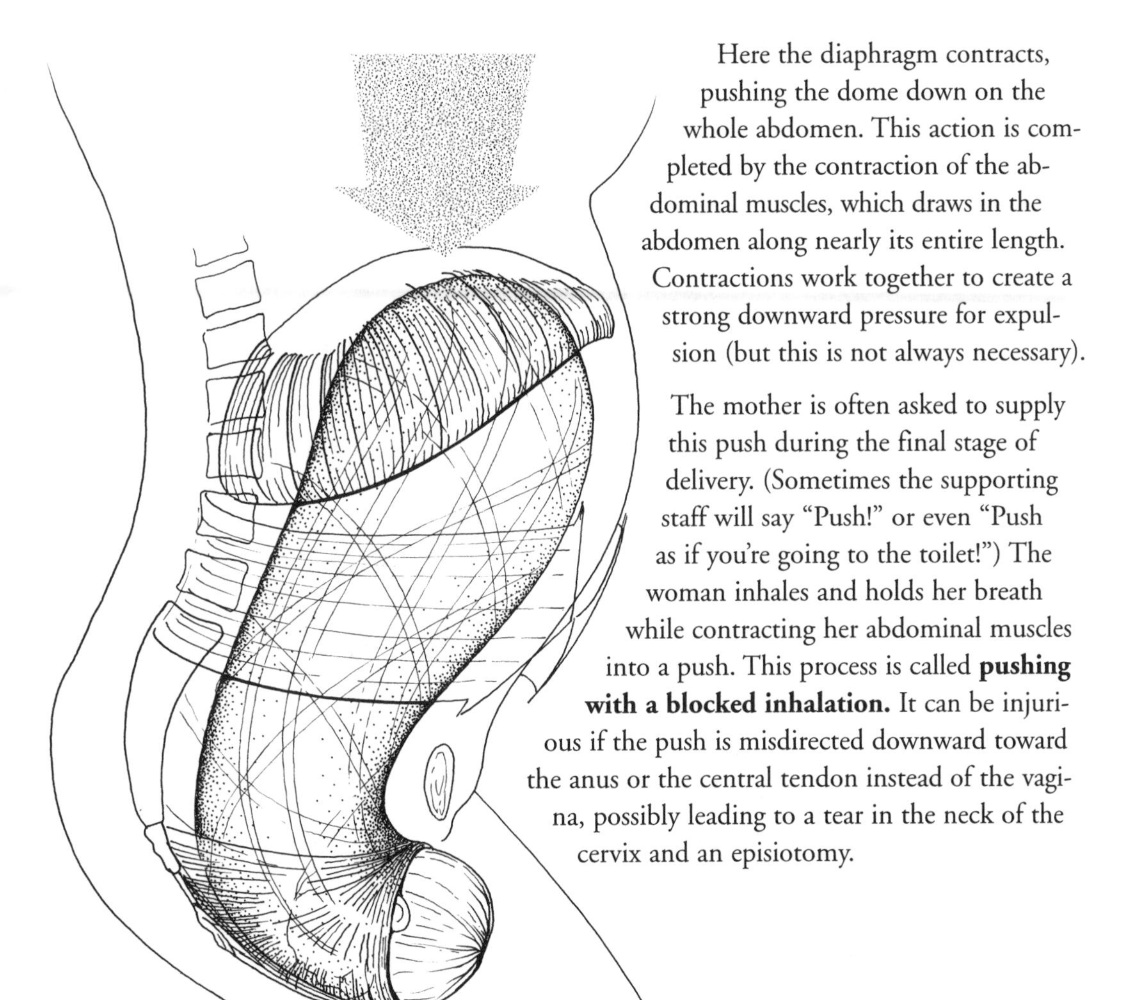

Here the diaphragm contracts, pushing the dome down on the whole abdomen. This action is completed by the contraction of the abdominal muscles, which draws in the abdomen along nearly its entire length. Contractions work together to create a strong downward pressure for expulsion (but this is not always necessary).

The mother is often asked to supply this push during the final stage of delivery. (Sometimes the supporting staff will say "Push!" or even "Push as if you're going to the toilet!") The woman inhales and holds her breath while contracting her abdominal muscles into a push. This process is called **pushing with a blocked inhalation.** It can be injurious if the push is misdirected downward toward the anus or the central tendon instead of the vagina, possibly leading to a tear in the neck of the cervix and an episiotomy.

This kind of pushing has its advantages and disadvantages.

Advantage: A push of such strength is *very efficient for expelling the baby* in the last stage of delivery, and is particularly advantageous when there is concern for the life of the fetus.

Disadvantages: On the other hand, *it can be too strong,* sometimes leading to an excessive amount of compression, which can damage the perineum, particularly its ligamentous structures. Alternatively, such an intense push can lead to a reflex reaction in the pelvic muscles, which are strongly stretched at this point. Instead of relaxing, the pelvic muscles can react by contracting, thereby increasing the risk of muscular injury and tears.

For these reasons, women are generally asked to *stop pushing when they start the second phase of stretching and opening of the perineum.* This helps avoid the superficial muscular tearing, but not the compulsory tearing of the deeper ligaments.

Why the diaphragm doesn't interfere when pushing during exhalation

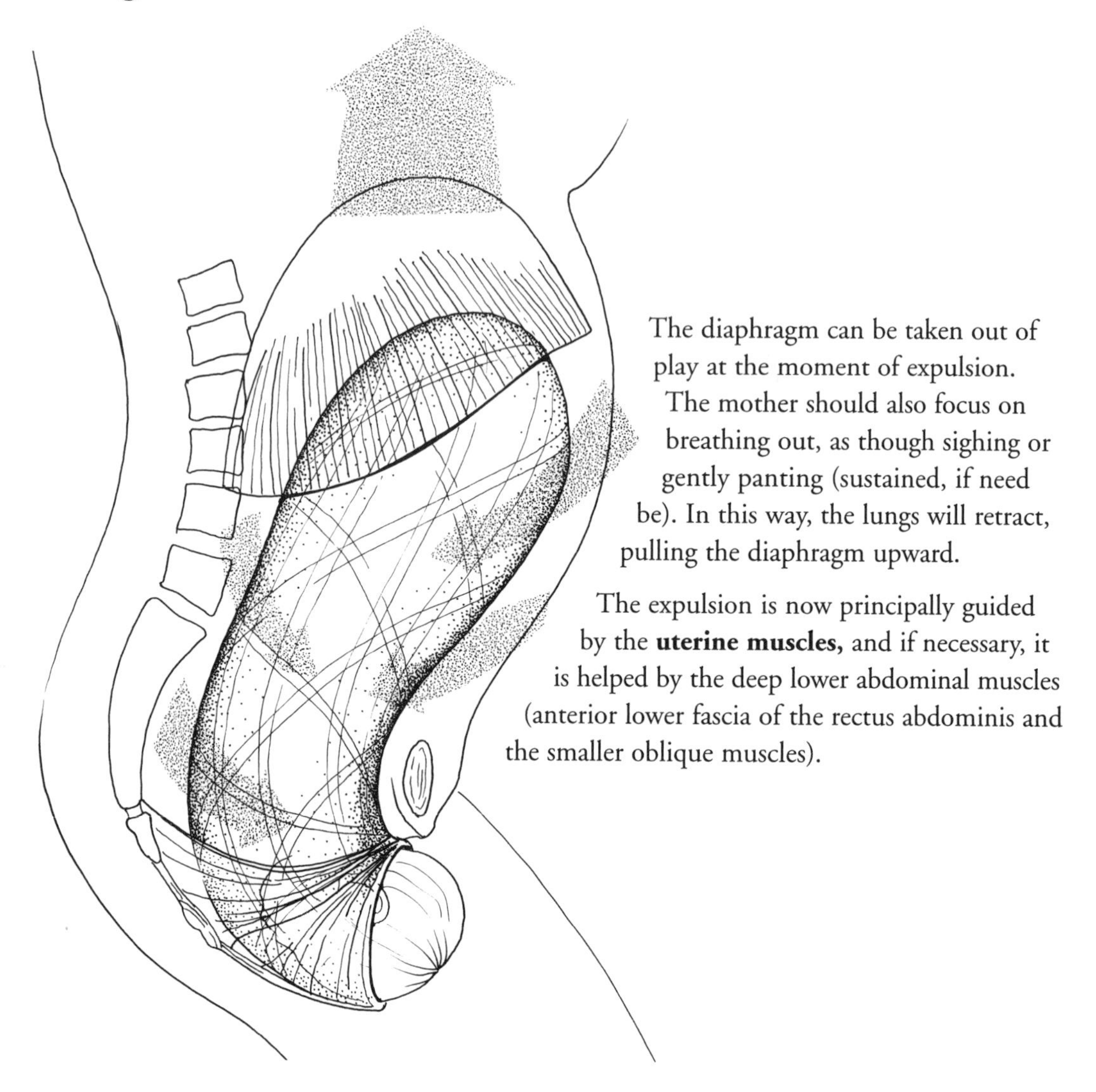

The diaphragm can be taken out of play at the moment of expulsion. The mother should also focus on breathing out, as though sighing or gently panting (sustained, if need be). In this way, the lungs will retract, pulling the diaphragm upward.

The expulsion is now principally guided by the **uterine muscles,** and if necessary, it is helped by the deep lower abdominal muscles (anterior lower fascia of the rectus abdominis and the smaller oblique muscles).

Once again, this mode of expulsion has its advantages and disadvantages.

Advantages: The *compression of the perineal muscles is far more gradual* and gives the muscles more time to relax. In addition, *the expulsive uterine push is more precisely directed* as it is much closer to the baby than that of the blocked inhalation push (discussed on the previous page), which is more peripheral. *The direction will be more clearly toward the vagina* and the anterior part of the perineum, and there will be less risk of tearing the central tendinous point of the perineum.

Disadvantages: If the unborn baby is at risk anyway, the blocked inspiration pushing method produces *faster results.*

If the uterus is in poor tone, as can happen if the mother is tired, either from before delivery or as a result of a long delivery, then the action of the uterus can be *coupled with that of the lower abdominal muscles,* which can help take up some of the slack.

CHAPTER FIVE

Analysis of Certain Movements

The following pages will show how certain movements engage the bones, joints, muscles, and organs. You will find that we often refer to these analyses in Chapter 8, *Exercises.*

In certain situations the pressure on the pelvis from the abdomen is increased

There are actions that put all the muscles of the perineum (those of the pelvic floor as well as the three orifices and their sphincters) into a resistance mode, i.e., *the muscles respond with intense contractions.* These actions are shown here with a score of one to four crosses, depending on whether they create a weak (+) or a very strong (++++) response.

The contents of the abdomen experience a sudden fall, dropping onto the pelvic floor, caused by:

- jumping (++++)
- running (+++)
- walking quickly (++).

All of these situations occur frequently in sports activities, particularly intense sport activities, which explains why the muscles of the perineum are put under stress.

The abdominal organs can exert pressure upon the muscles of the perineum by:

- Squatting, with the thighs compressing the abdomen (see p. 79). This is considerably accentuated by the presence of abdominal fat (+++).
- Wearing tight clothing, e.g., belts or tight jeans, can put pressure on the abdomen, which has repercussions for the perineum (++).
- Excessive reinforcement of the abdominal walls. A highly toned abdominal musculature (found in women athletes with highly developed muscles) can, paradoxically, compress the perineum, especially if the exercise reinforces the abdominal wall at the waist level, producing an hour-glass figure (++). (Alternative methods of reinforcing the abdominals are described on pp. 118-121.)

The diaphragm can exert pressure on the abdominal contents, just as it does on the abdominal muscles, when bearing down (from + to ++++) during:

- urination
- delivery
- defecation.

In addition, extra pressure can result in heavy weight-bearing when bracing the abdomen, or alternatively, when the legs are called upon to make extra efforts, as in climbing stairs (+).

The abdomen can be compressed upward by the abdominal muscles. If this happens suddenly, part of the pressure will be directed downward, compressing the pelvic floor, e.g.:

- speaking loudly (+) or shouting (++)
- blowing with effort, e.g., blowing up a balloon (+++) or blowing out candles (++)
- laughing loudly (++)
- coughing (people with chronic coughing or chronic bronchitis often have distended or overworked abdominal muscles) (++++)
- vomiting (+++)
- sneezing (++++).

In all these situations, there is:

- a strong risk of urinary leakage
- increased risk of prolapse (see pp. 90-93).

However, these particular actions can also be turned to your advantage to provoke more intense exercising of the perineum, especially as these are ordinary, everyday occurrences, rather than formal exercises. For this reason, they are encouraged in Chapter 8 as advanced level coordination and integration exercises (see pp. 135-138). *These exercises should not be taken up if leakage from the vaginal orifice or prolapse already exists, as they could make matters worse. In such cases, a physician should be consulted first.*

The squatting position

Squatting is a useful position for certain phases of childbirth and for exercising the perineum and certain internal organs. We will therefore discuss it in detail.

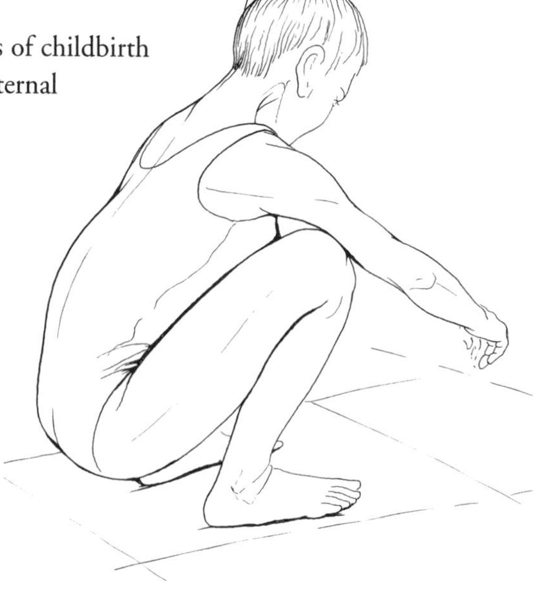

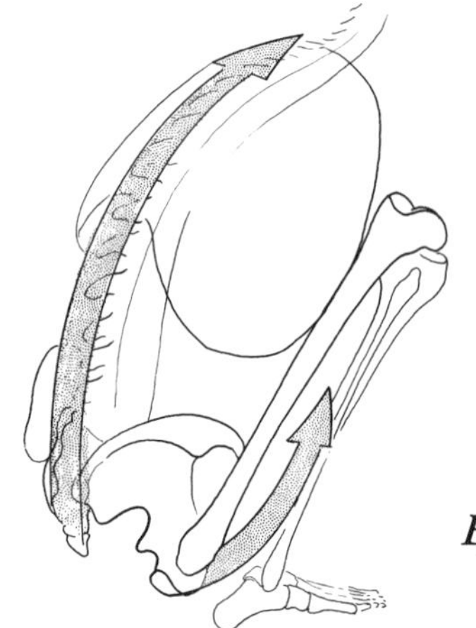

Effect on the pelvis

Because of the flexed position of the thighs and hips while squatting, the ilium bones are forced to strongly rotate posteriorly. In order to balance, the trunk is flexed forward. This stretches the posterior muscles of the trunk, which then hold the sacrum backward and prevent it from accompanying the ilium bones. As the coccyx is held back, the ischia move forward. This corresponds to a nutation of the sacrum and a widening of the inferior opening.

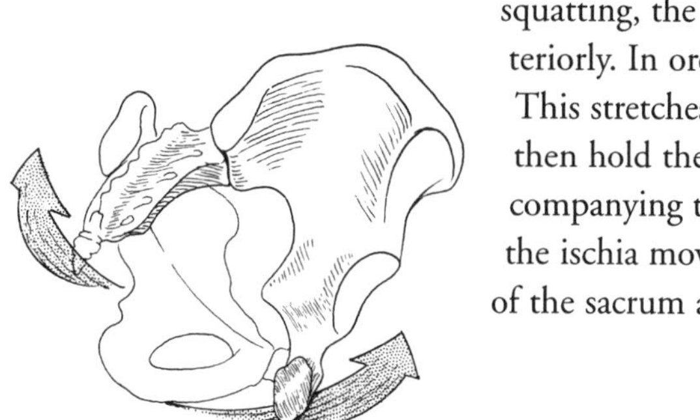

Effect on the perineum

The perineum is put under tension from front to back, stretching the skin and the muscular layers. This should be taken into account as you formulate a mental image of this area while maintaining this position (see p. 112). In addition, the stretching of the muscles will induce a corresponding reflex action, i.e., a contraction.

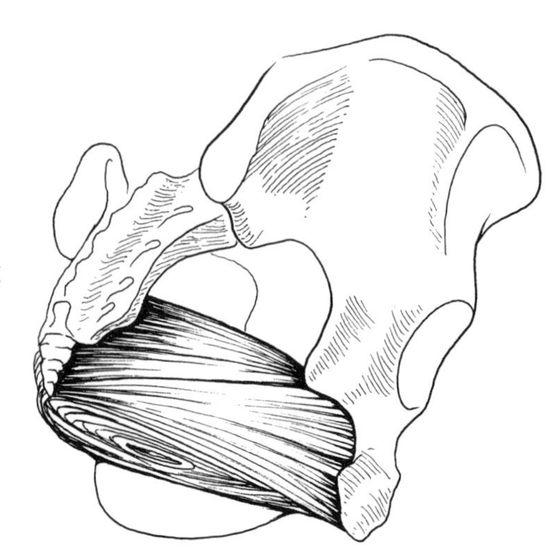

Effect on the abdominal contents

Compressed by the thighs, the abdomen is pushed:

- backward
  - partly upward
  - partly downward

and as a result, the abdomen exerts pressure on the perineum.

This added pressure could be used to increase the resistance of the perineum (see p. 112).

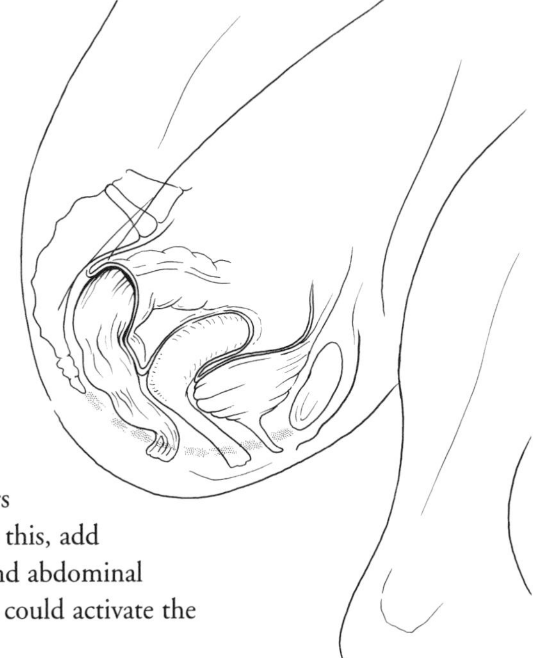

Effect on the organs of the lesser pelvis

The affected organs include:

- the bladder, which is compressed by the abdomen, and the urethra, which is stretched. The result is an urge to urinate.
- the vagina, which is ready for the bearing down needed in delivery
- the rectum, which is mobilized and appears compressed from the back to the front. To this, add the stretching of the posterior perineum and abdominal compression toward the back, all of which could activate the defecation reflex.

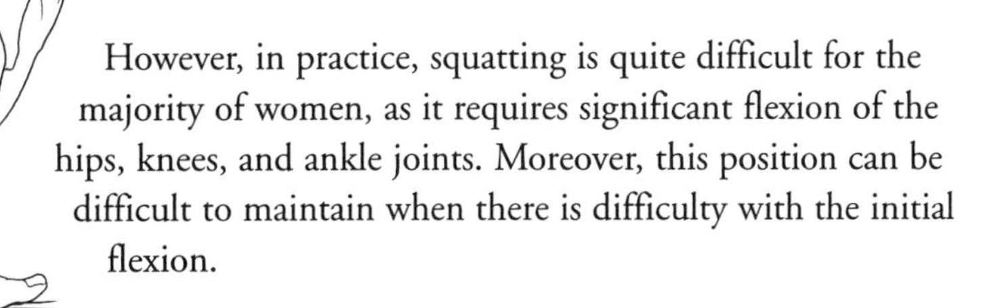

However, in practice, squatting is quite difficult for the majority of women, as it requires significant flexion of the hips, knees, and ankle joints. Moreover, this position can be difficult to maintain when there is difficulty with the initial flexion.

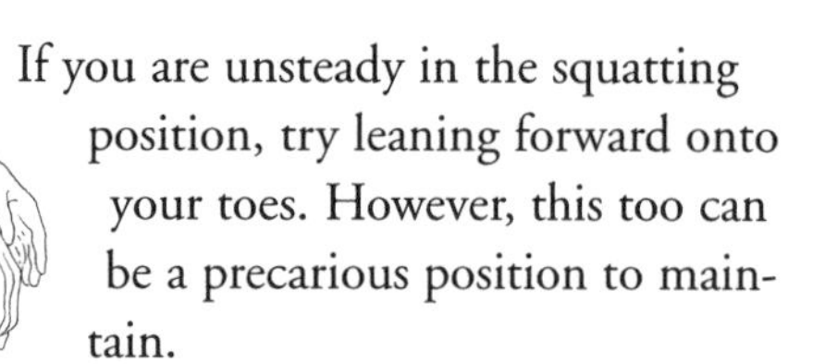

If you are unsteady in the squatting position, try leaning forward onto your toes. However, this too can be a precarious position to maintain.

If it is unavoidable, you should help support yourself in the following ways to perform the exercises described in this book:

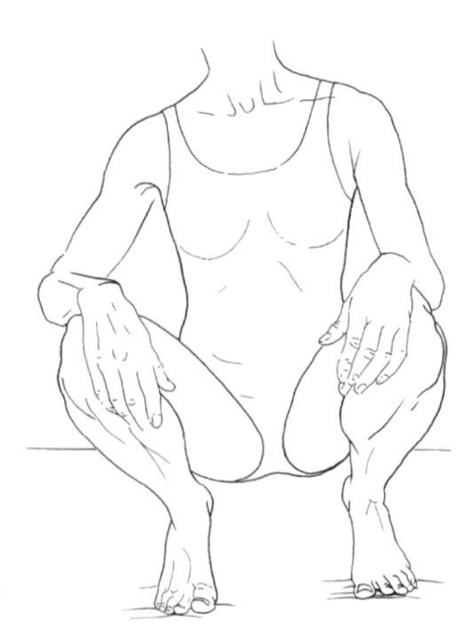

Raise the heels (by a few centimeters).

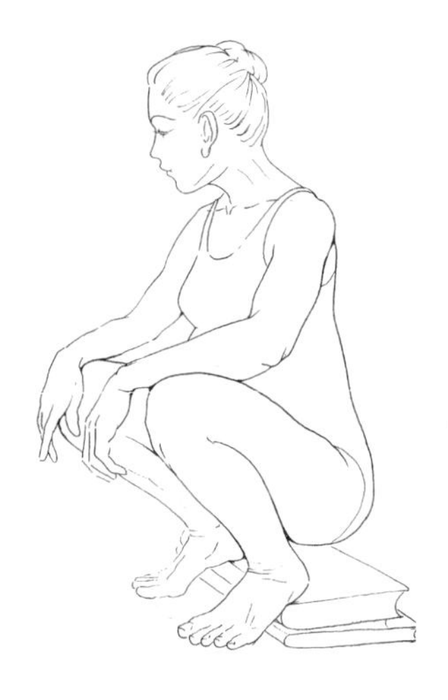

Lean forward against a support.

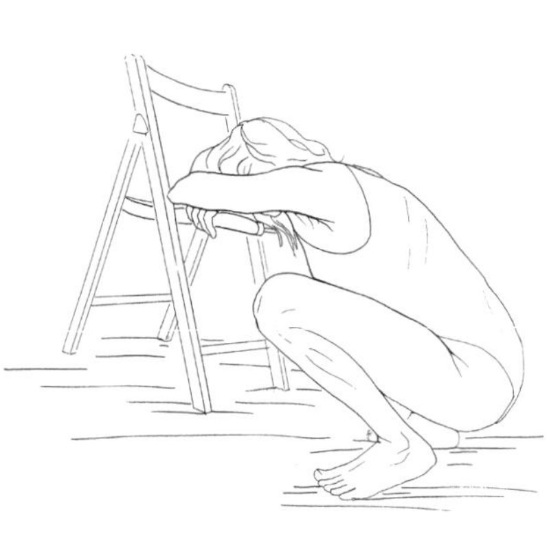

Lean backward against a support.

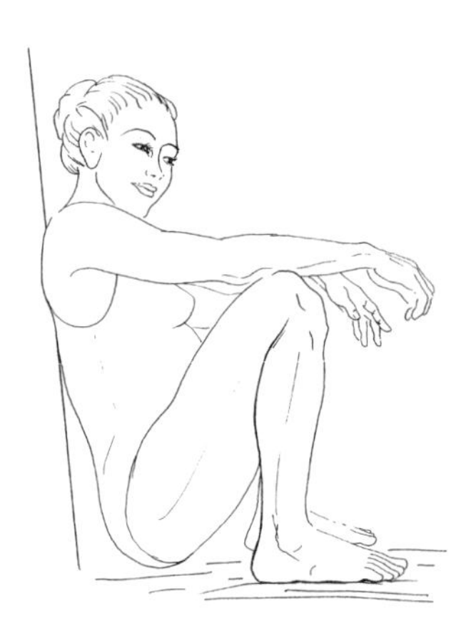

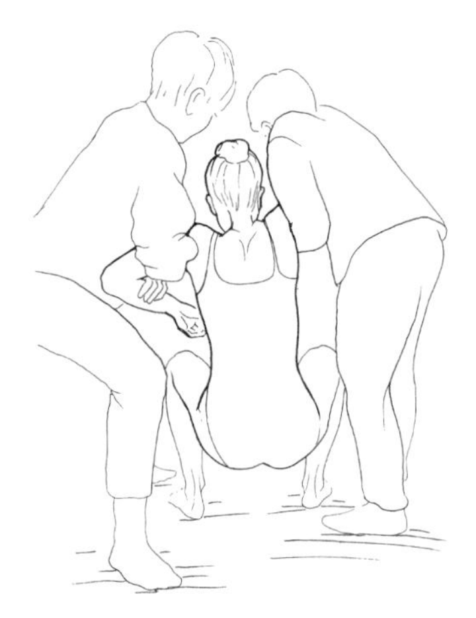

On the day of the delivery, have two people support you. This supported squatting position has two advantages:

- As the shoulders are lifted they pull up the ribs, and with them the diaphragm, which then exerts less pressure on the uterus.
- By being suspended there is less compression on the legs; this improves the venous circulation, since it is less impeded.

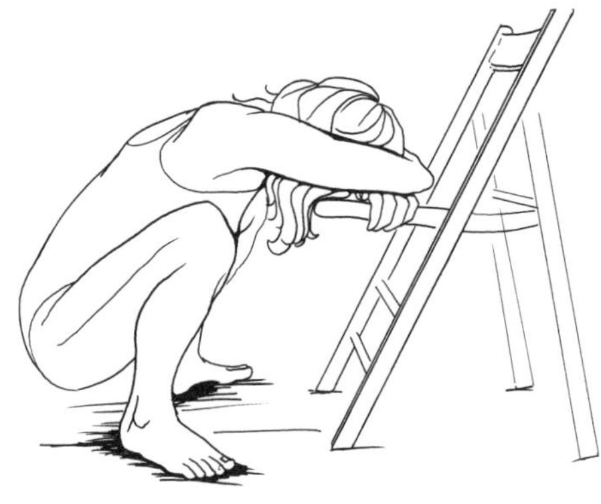

How the position of the thighs changes the relationships in the bony pelvis

When we change the position of the thighs, we modify the angle of flexion at the hip joints and put tension on the muscles and ligaments. This increased tension will rock the ilium bones.

Hyperflexed thighs

Increased tension in the ligaments and muscles of the hip joints will bring about a posterior rotation of the ilium bones. The ischia move forward, opening up the inferior rim (which is useful for the bearing-down phase of childbirth).

Moderately flexed thighs

In this position, the anterior and posterior ligaments and muscles are relaxed and the ilium bones are free to move forward or backward (anterior and posterior rotation, respectively; see pp. 30 and 31).

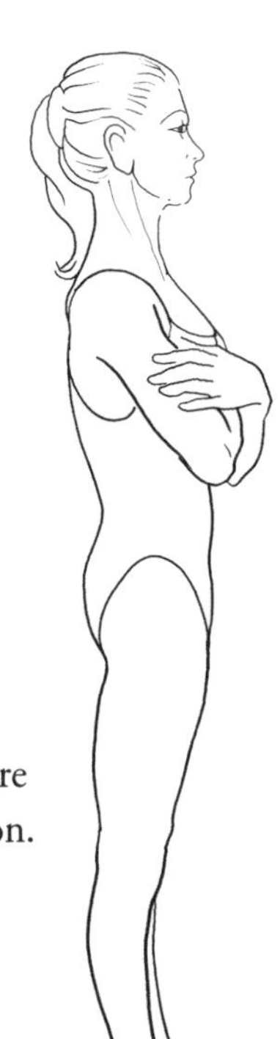

Extended thighs

The ilium bones are pulled forward (anterior rotation). However, when you are lying down, the sacrum cannot move against the ground to follow this rotation. As a result, only the ilium bones are able to move.

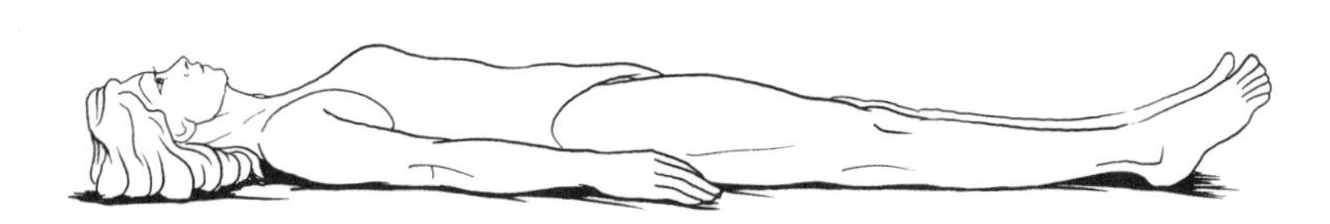

Examples of positions and postures for both the day of delivery and pelvic floor exercises

The positions and postures presented here are useful in many different ways, both for the day of delivery and as cues for doing exercises for the perineum. They can be used after the exercises in Chapter 8 have been assimilated in order to expand the number of ways that those exercises can be performed.

For each of these positions, the following analysis will be applied:

- Is the pelvis pulled into anterior or posterior rotation?
- Is the pelvis free to move between anterior and posterior rotation?
- Is the sacrum pulled into nutation or counter-nutation?
- During delivery, does the weight factor influence the expulsion of the fetus in a downward direction, and during exercises of the perineum, does it increase pressure on the perineum?

Here, "weight (+)" indicates that the weight factor has an effect, while "weight (-)" indicates that it does not.

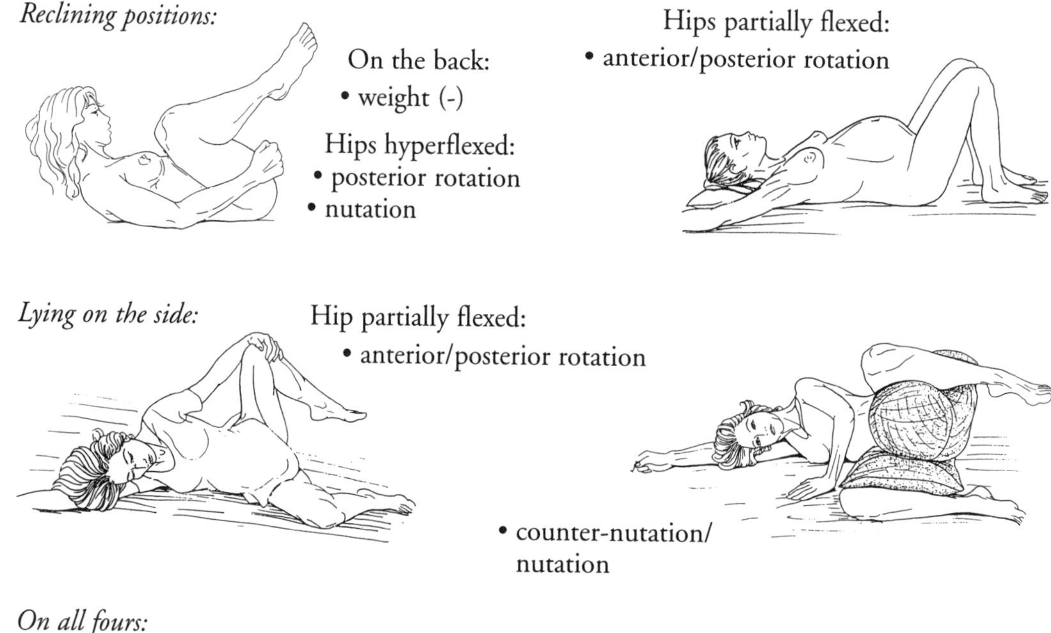

On all fours:

Back horizontal:
- weight (-)
- anterior/posterior rotation
- counter-nutation/ nutation

With the back leaning forward:
- weight (--)
- posterior rotation
- nutation

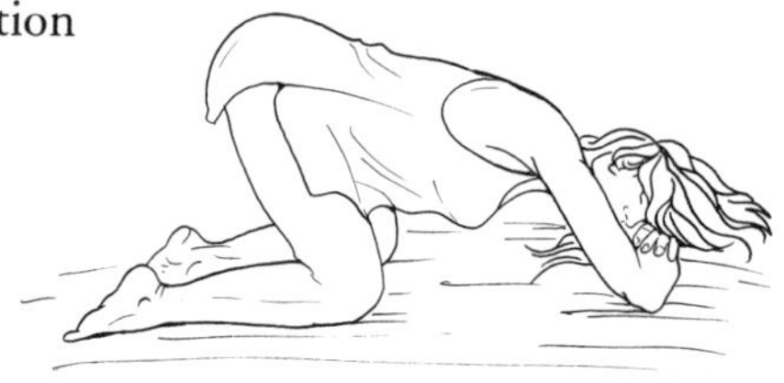

Sitting positions:

Leaning forward or backward:
- weight (+)

Hips partially flexed (far right):
- anterior/posterior rotation
- counter-nutation/nutation

Hips hyperflexed (below right):
- posterior rotation
- nutation

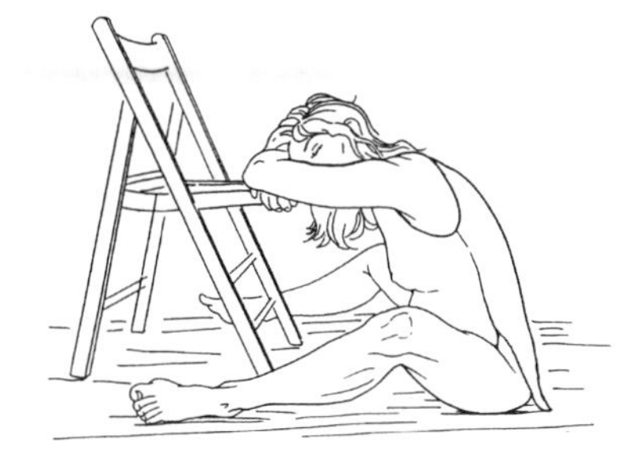

Squatting position:

Hips partially flexed:
- weight (+)
- posterior rotation
- nutation

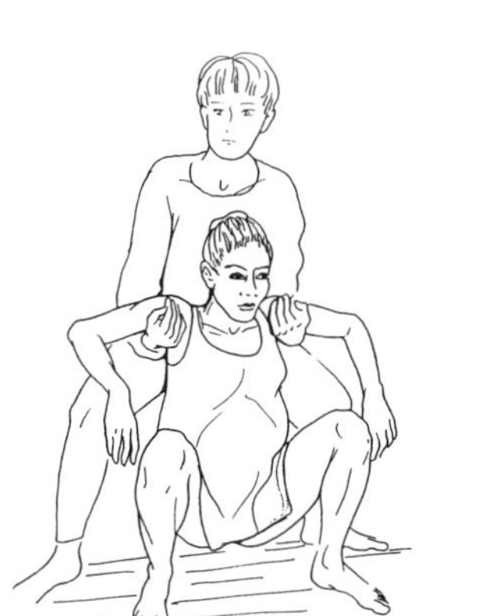

Standing Positions:

Hips partially flexed:
- (weight +)
- anterior/posterior rotation
- counter-nutation/ nutation

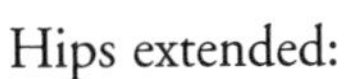

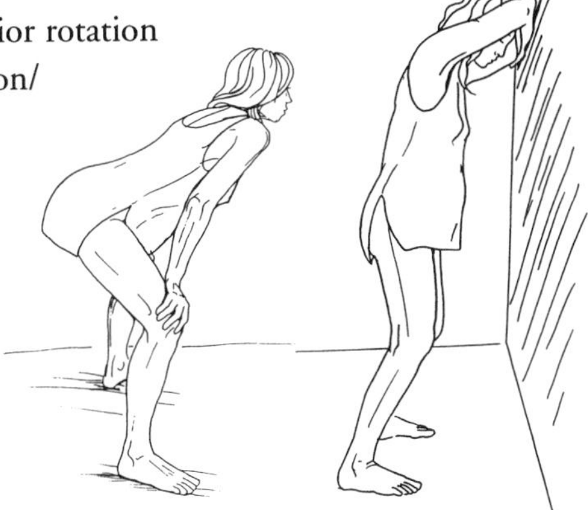

Hips extended:
- weight (+)
- anterior rotation
- counter-nutation

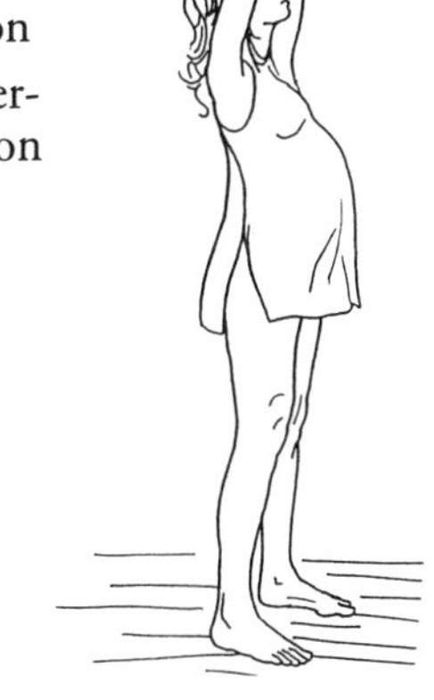

Get to know these positions. Try them out yourself—both during pregnancy and during exercises for the perineum—and experiment with them. Learn about the anatomical effects on the pelvis and internal organs when you choose different postures. Doing these things will enable you to choose the position that is best suited to the different stages of childbirth, or to the perineal exercise that you wish to perform.

CHAPTER SIX

The Perineum and Delivery

The culmination of the complex process that enables the fetus to leave the mother's body is called delivery. Naturally, the child is the main focus of this event. However, the final stage when the baby is expelled from the uterus—expulsion—can put the mother's perineum under considerable strain.

For this reason, the brief description provided here focuses particularly on the perineal region. For a more detailed account, we recommend, especially for pregnant women, Frederik Leboyer's book, *Birth Without Violence.*

The two stages of delivery

First stage

The first stage, called **dilation,** begins with a recognizable series of contractions of the uterus. The contractions are rhythmic and regular, and grow more and more intense. They are separated by moments of complete relaxation that become shorter as labor proceeds.

The contractions occur throughout the uterus, from the top to the cervix. To begin with, the cervix is thick and closed. The contractions will progressively bring about a dilation of the cervix to the point where it becomes completely eliminated as the uterus opens right out into the vagina, which is also dilated. The time this takes is variable, ranging from one to many hours.

Contractions push the baby downward, past the upper rim and into the pelvic cavity (see pp. 19 and 21). This process is called **engagement.** (Engagement here is different from the same term used near the end of pregnancy when the the baby moves toward the pelvis, a reversible movement. Here engagement describes the entrance of the baby into the bony circle of the pelvic cavity, as shown on p. 25.) If the head engages first, it will then turn, accommodating its size to that of the pelvic cavity (see pp. 26 and 27). It will then pass through the middle and lower pelvic rims.

Second stage

Finally, the head comes to rest against the last passageway which it must traverse—the perineum. This marks the second stage of delivery, or **expulsion.** The pressure of the head on the pelvic floor brings about a reflex contraction of the uterus, the **expulsive reflex** (see p. 71). The mother usually feels an urge to push, and the uterine contractions become almost uncontrollable. Pressure from the head as well as from the contractions cause the perineum to stretch, in two phases: first posteriorly, and then anteriorly. These changes are the final events of labor before the delivery and will be described on the next page.

How the perineum stretches during labor (in expulsion)

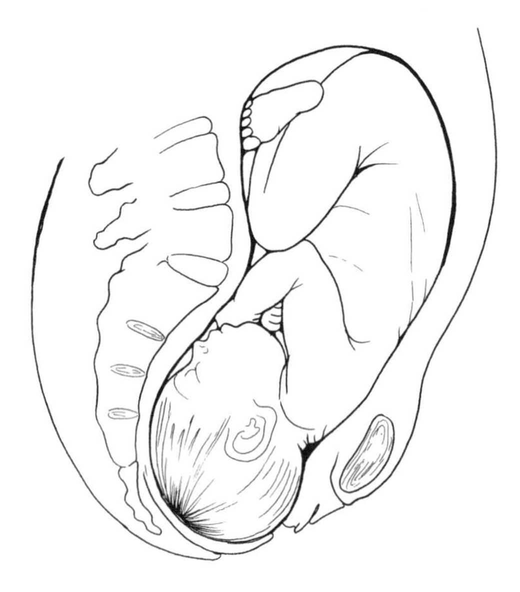

First of all the baby passes downward, moving obliquely and toward the back, along the sacrum.

The baby's head reaches the coccyx, which it pushes toward the back, pushing the anal region outward and opening the anal orifice. This is referred to as the **expansion of the posterior perineum.**

However, the movement of the coccyx in the posterior direction is soon limited.

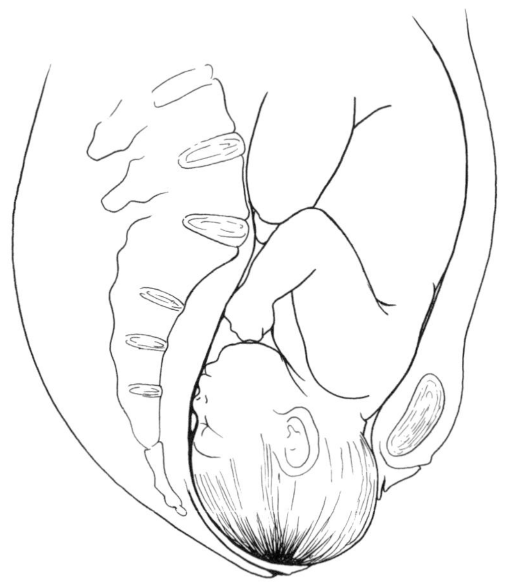

At this point, the second phase, i.e., the **expansion of the anterior perineum,** begins.

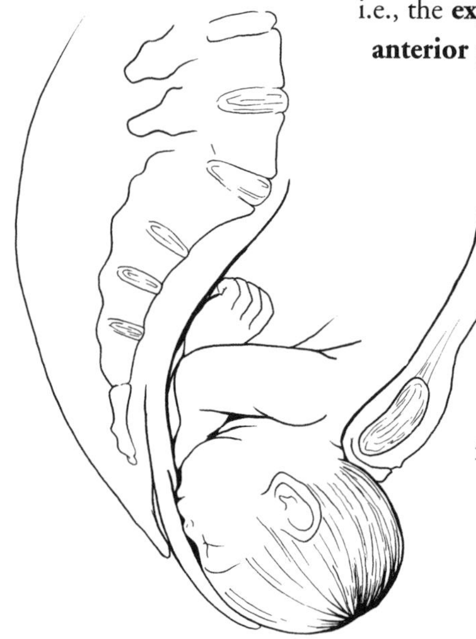

The baby's head is pushed toward the front, along the concave surface of the sacrum. It passes through the **urogenital hiatus** in front (see p. 40) and stretches out the anterior perineum, which in turn bulges outward as well. The distance between the anus and the vulva increases during this expansion from three to eight centimeters.

The different types of presentations

The term **presentation** refers to that part of the baby which, at the moment of delivery, lies over the pelvic brim.

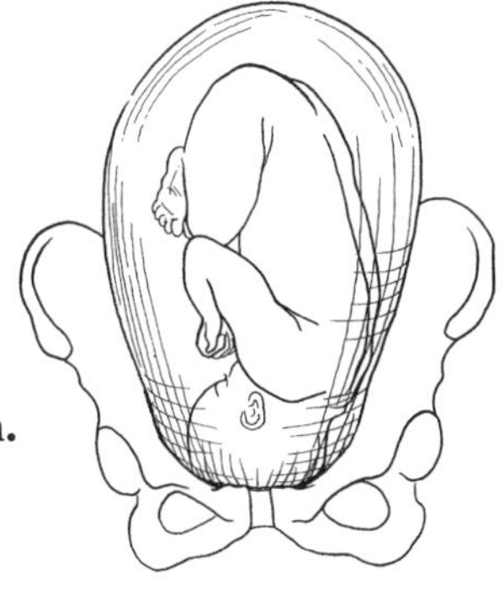

In most cases, the baby presents with head first, which is called a **vertex presentation.**

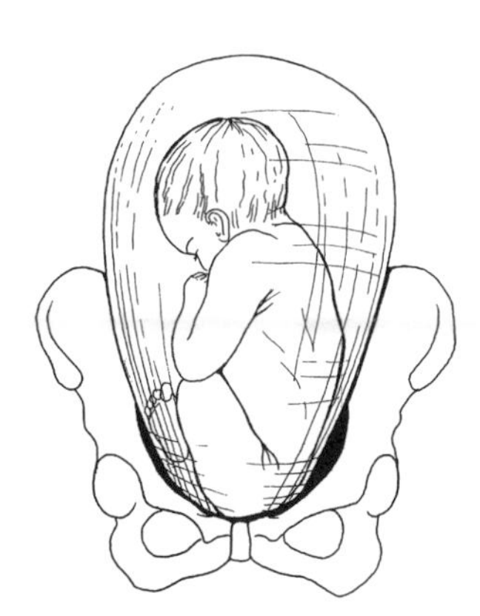

Less frequently, the baby presents with the bottom first, which is called a **breech presentation.**

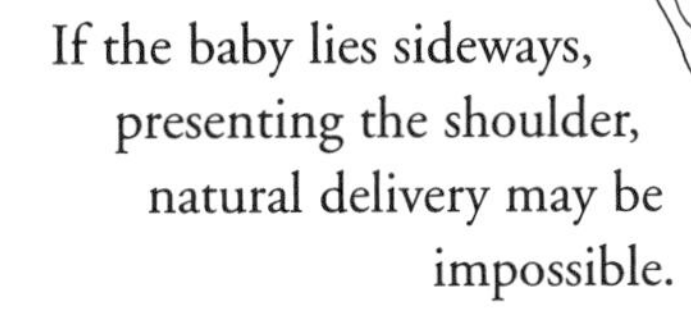

If the baby lies sideways, presenting the shoulder, natural delivery may be impossible.

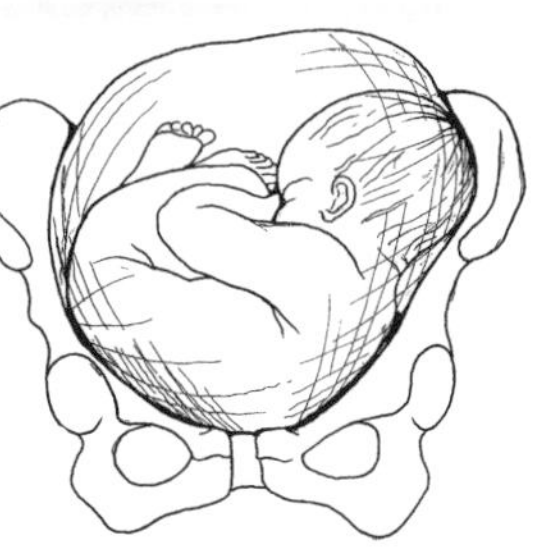

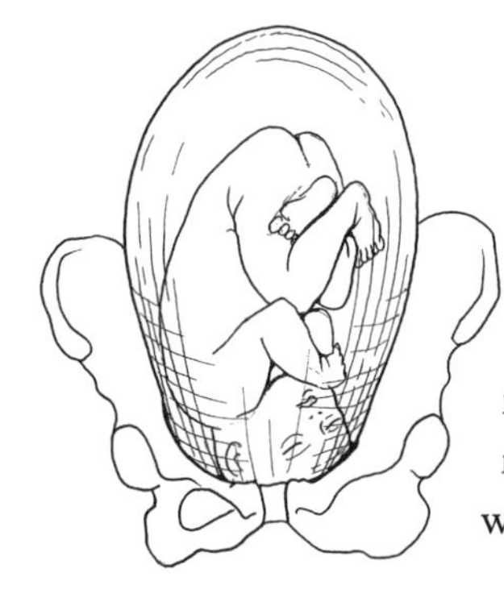

Each of these three presentations has its own variants, especially the vertex presentation, where the baby's head may engage facing the sacrum (as described on the previous page) or the pubis. In the case of the latter presentation, the largest aspect of the head (see p. 27) moves toward the perineum during the delivery. This delivery is more difficult for the baby and also for the mother, whose perineum will be over-distended.

In fact, toward the end of the pregnancy, positions taken up by the mother can influence the position of the baby and the way in which it becomes engaged in the pelvis. In forward-leaning (and upright) positions, the baby turns around with its back lying as though in a hammock against the mother's abdomen, and its head turned toward the mother's back. The baby will start the delivery with its head turned toward the sacrum, and the back of its head will be presented toward the vulva. This is the best position.

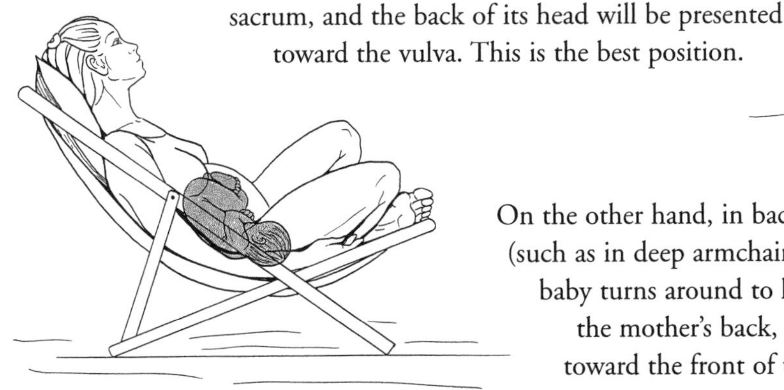

On the other hand, in backward-lying positions (such as in deep armchairs or deckchairs), the baby turns around to lie with its back against the mother's back, and its head turned toward the front of the abdomen.

If it engages in this way, the baby will pass through the birth canal with its head turned toward the pubis and its forehead or face turned toward the vulva. This is a less favorable position.

Injury that can occur to the perineum during delivery

Injury can occur as a result of multiple deliveries, the baby's birthweight, or, most importantly, aspects of the delivery itself, e.g.:

- a rapid or lengthy delivery
- more than eight intense blocked-breath pushes (see p. 73) without the use of the expulsive reflex (see p. 71)
- manual pressure upon the uterus.

These factors, especially in combination, can impede the natural perineal stretching and cause muscular tearing or collapse. If an episiotomy is performed too late or improperly, injury will not be avoided.

During the final phase of delivery (the expulsion), it is important that the mother stop pushing and that the midwife:

- support the perineum
- allow the baby's head to turn and disengage
- perform an episiotomy if necessary, and in a timely fashion!

The tissues at risk include:

- ligaments, especially the round ligament and the uterosacral ligaments, which are already overstretched as a result of the pregnancy (see p. 57)
- adhering surfaces, such as the vesicovaginal (or Halban's) fascia between the bladder and the vagina (see p. 48)
- aponeurotic surfaces, such as the perineal membrane (see pp. 37 and 54)
- muscles, especially the sphincter muscles (which can be "crushed" when the baby's head is delivered), the muscles of the pelvic floor (which may have been torn), and the puborectalis bundle of the levator ani (see p. 40)
- fibrous nucleus of the central tendon of the perineum (see p. 42).

CHAPTER SEVEN

Some Pathologies Common to the Lesser Pelvis

Pathologies of the lower pelvis vary according to which of the three different systems they belong: urinary, genital, or digestive. The following pages describe frequent disorders related to the three organs within this region

Note: All the descriptions here are of a general nature. *They are not a substitute for a diagnosis, which is the domain of a physician.* Some of the exercises on the practice pages could be of use in relation to certain pathologies, *but should not be practiced without first consulting your physician.*

The disorders of the lower pelvis described here are of three kinds:

- difficulty with the retention of urine or feces (**incontinence**) or the opposite, an over-retention (**continence**)
- the falling of an organ from its usual position (**prolapse** or **ptosis**)
- breakdown of motor reflexes between the different organs.

These three different pathologies can be cumulative, and the onset of one can provoke the occurrence of the others as well.

Urinary incontinence

This can be defined as the inablity to voluntarily control the outflow of urine. There are a number of different causes and manifestations of this condition. We will discuss only the most frequent ones here.

Incontinence of effort

This is an involuntary loss of urine as a result of an increase in abdominal pressure (see p. 76). It can occur regardless of how full the bladder might be, but it is more likely to happen when the bladder is full.

Incontinence of effort is often the result of a lack of muscle tone, particularly of the support muscles, e.g., the urethral sphincter. It frequently occurs during the last phase of pregnancy and during the weeks following delivery. The condition will normally disappear, but it may stay or reappear during menopause as a result of loss of muscular strength linked to hormonal changes. Some women are more at risk than others to this type of incontinence because of their particular circumstances or lifestyle, such as those who suffer from prolonged coughing attacks (as in chronic bronchitis), or, paradoxically, athletes engaged in intense training programs. Many sports that involve running, jumping, or bouncing can provoke rapid and repeated changes in abdominal pressure on the perineum. If you suffer from sudden incontinence, try doing, for a few weeks, the exercises recommended for identifying and strengthening the pelvic floor muscles (see pp.108-117), and those for the bladder and the urethra (pp. 126-129).

If the incontinence persists, the cause may not be muscular and a medical diagnosis will be necessary together with more specialized treatment, such as physical therapy. After the delivery of your baby, an assessment of the condition of the pelvic floor will normally be given, together with proposed treatment (if necessary), which should help to avoid any future incontinence.

Incontinence as a result of an unstable bladder

As we have seen, urination is an involuntary act, a reflex action of the bladder muscle triggered by the urge to urinate. This occurs when the bladder reaches a certain degree of fullness. In adults, the first sensation occurs when the volume of fluid in the bladder is approximately 200 milliliters, and there is a sense of urgency when the volume reaches 400-500 milliliters.

Sometimes, an intense and even painful sense of urgency can occur with a volume of only 150-200 milliliters, possibly as a result of contractions of the bladder that occur too quickly and too often. This would be a hyperactive or unstable bladder condition, and could result in highly irregular urination, depending on the following responses of the urethral sphincter:

- When there is sufficient contraction, continence is assured, but the need to urinate occurs too frequently. This is called **urinary urgency.**
- When there is insufficient contraction of the sphincter, resulting in partial incontinence, it is called **stress incontinence.**
- When there is no contraction at all, there is **total incontinence.** This occurs because of a disturbance in the urinary reflex. This is very common among the elderly (where the functioning of the nervous system is altered), but it can also occur in younger people.

It is important to note that all three of these conditions can have other causes, which are not described here.

If you suffer from the urgent or frequent need to urinate, you can try the exercises for bladder and urethral control described on pp.126-129. These exercises may help you to restore the natural urinary cycle of reflexes and response. If your problem is not helped by these exercises, you should seek a medical diagnosis and treatment.

Urinary retention

Normally, the bladder empties completely after urination. Under certain conditions, however, it will only partially empty, or empty too infrequently, even though urine produced in the kidneys continues to flow through the ureters. There are a number of reasons why this might happen: atonal bladder; imprecise perception of the pressure; a habit of "holding in," leading to retention; an obstacle in the urethral tract (e.g., stone, narrowing of the urethra, or cancer) or bladder.

In the latter case, the bladder may have to work against resistance, which would considerably thicken the bladder muscle. This is called a **stressed bladder.**

Vaginal prolapse

The vagina can become stretched or lacking in muscle tone. In such cases, the vulva bulges out, with the inner lips stretched apart (when normally they should be touching), and the entry to the vagina opens abnormally wide. This may give rise to the sound of escaping vaginal air (which has entered the vagina and is expelled during certain kinds of compression movement), or allow water from the bath to enter the vagina, which then leads to vaginal leakage of water after the bath. For any of these conditions, try the exercises for the vagina described on pp. 129-131.

Vaginismus

In this condition, the vagina is excessively contracted, resulting in discomfort or even pain during sexual intercourse. (Difficult or painful coitus is called **dyspareunia**). There are a number of causes, including lesions during delivery, problems of intravaginal secretions, or psychological problems. The exercises recommended on pp. 129-131 will eventually help correct the problem. Pay special attention to the exercises that promote relaxation and breathing between contractions.

Fecal incontinence

This occurs when the feces cannot be retained. It is a problem that may be encountered after delivery. There are a variety of causes, the most common of which are:

- The rectum may have insufficient capacity.
- The rectum may contract too often.
- The ability to contract strongly may be lacking at the level of the striated sphincter of the anus, as well as in the muscles of the pelvic floor that surround the lower rectum and close the anal orifice (see p. 61).

Terminal constipation

In this type of constipation, the pathology concerns the rectum, the last part of the large intestine. There are many causes, including:

- distended or not very contractile rectum
- lack of relaxation by sphincter muscles.

These two pathologies, which appear to be opposites, can result from *pushing during a blocked inhalation,* a method that is used to help expel the baby during delivery (see p. 73). This process involves contractions of the diaphragm and abdominal muscles, resulting in pushing the perineum (and the baby). However, excessively strong contractions of the diaphragm and abdominal muscles can result in the following events:

- prolapse of the organs, especially of the rectum, which is the most easily stretched
- excessive stretching of the levator ani and sphincter muscles
- stretching of the nerve supply to these muscles, resulting in neuromotor degradation.

Each of these factors can cause incontinence. Some instances of terminal constipation can be improved through exercise of the rectum and anus (see pp. 132-135).

Prolapse

A **prolapsed organ** is one which has dropped or descended partially or completely (in this case from the lower pelvis) as a result of deterioration or slackening in its means of support. Of concern to us are prolapses of the:

- *Vagina.* When the vagina descends, the downward collapse of the vaginal wall is called a **vaginocele.**
- *Uterus.* The uterus can descend partially or completely into the vagina, which is known as **uterine prolapse.** In a first degree prolapse, the cervix is still clearly in the vagina. In a second degree prolapse, it can descend to the end of the vagina. And in a third degree prolapse, the cervix protrudes from the body. The uterus can pull the bladder with it as it descends, and the bladder will then protrude into the front wall of the vagina, making the anterior surface bulge (**cystocele**).
- *Rectum.* The rectum can also be pulled downward into the vagina, making its posterior surface bulge (**rectocele**). In addition, the rectum can slip down upon itself and protrude outside the anus, pulling the anus with it and resulting in:
  - —an **anal prolapse,** when only the anal skin descends
  - —a **rectal prolapse,** when the interior wall of the rectum descends.
- *Peritoneum.* The peritoneum in the region of the pouch of Douglas can be pulled into the vagina, which will also make the posterior surface bulge, forming a colpocele.

In the latter three conditions, the extent of the descent of each organ can vary considerably. The bladder, rectum, and peritoneum can drop a little or a lot, to the extent of protruding into the opening of the vagina. In addition, the different types of prolapse can be cumulative, and the symptoms can vary as well. At first, there may be a feeling of heaviness in the region of the vagina, or a gaping feeling at the level of the vulva that worsens during moments of intense intraabdominal pressure. *If you recognize any of these symptoms or sensations, consult your physician.*

The treatment for a prolapse varies, depending upon its importance. Every treatment should be based on a medical diagnosis and be given under medical supervision. Certain relatively mild prolapses can sometimes be improved by the exercises described in this book. Of particular importance are those exercises that take pressure off the organs through specific breathing techniques (see p. 135), as well as those that strengthen the pelvic floor (pp. 108-117), except, of course, for those exercises that put any pressure on the perineum.

You can also seek help from specialized physiotherapists in the reeducation of the affected muscles. It may be recommended that a **pesary** be put in place. A pesary is a soft ring that, when placed around the cervix, can prevent the uterus from descending further into the vagina. Where a prolapse is more advanced or uncomfortable, surgery is often the best answer.

Hemorrhoids

A **hemorrhoid** is one or more distended veins situated in swollen tissue in the rectum wall. It can distend within or outside the rectum and cause various complications. A woman may often experience hemorrhoids for the first time after her delivery, or the delivery may exacerbate a previous condition. During labor, as the fetus descends, it exerts increasing pressure on the blood vessels of the lesser pelvis. In the final phase of delivery, the baby's head stretches the posterior perineum and compresses and pushes everything surrounding it toward the anus, including any blood that is located at that moment within the rectal veins. This will cause the veins to become distended. This same intense pressure persists through the entire final phase of disengagement of the baby.

The treatment of hemorrhoids requires medical care. At the same time, some simple rules of hygiene will help prevent them. Especially during pregnancy, the following are to be avoided:

- sitting too long without moving the legs, especially on soft surfaces
- long hot baths
- constipation.

You can do the following:

- Do the exercises to tone up the perineal muscles (see pp. 108-117 and 134), which stimulate the blood circulation in that area. Try to practice them a few times a day, especially when you must remain seated over long periods of time (e.g., during car, train, or plane trips).
- Do the breathing exercises on pp. 135-138 to take pressure off the lower pelvis.

CHAPTER EIGHT

Exercises

Important Precautions

This section of the book provides a series of exercises aimed at sensory and functional discovery, with training through repetition. The objective of the exercises is *in no way therapeutic,* although the exercises may be included in therapeutic programs. Rather, the objective is uniquely one of promoting health and the art of living. If the exercises had a therapeutic objective, it would be necessary to adapt them for different pathological conditions, diagnoses, and medical indications and contraindications. That is not the purpose of this book.

Certain exercises proposed here may be unsuitable for women with pathological conditions, or during a particular phase of life. Before starting this section, it is therefore essential that you review the brief summary of pathologies that are common to the lower pelvis in Chapter 7, as well as the precautions in Chapter 9, to determine which exercises are appropriate for you. In general, anyone undergoing treatment for lumbago, sciatica, cardiovascular disease, cancer, or neurological or psychological illness is advised to check with their physician before engaging in these exercises.

The practical work proposed here is directed at active body awareness based on a knowledge of the body's anatomy. As you approach each of the exercises, consider the following stages:

• **Form an accurate mental image of the body structures as you work with them.** At each stage there are *practical suggestions* that refer back to earlier chapters on the related anatomy. You should begin with a good understanding of the body part, organ, or muscle, and be able to form a clear mental image for yourself before starting the corresponding practical work.

• **Get a clear sensation before putting the muscle to work.** Each section begins with exercises to awaken the senses through a progressive discovery of the sensations associated with the movements of the bones, individual muscle layers, and the functions of various organs and their sphincters. You will learn to recognise and "train" them. Take the time to establish this *range of sensations* in yourself. It will be time well-spent, and will later serve to focus your practice so that the exercises are performed with precision.

• **Vary the quality of the muscular actions.** In these exercises the contraction of a muscle can serve different purposes: to discover a hitherto unknown muscle, to assess its strength (which is as important as its flexibility), or, conversely, its ability to relax. In addition, you will learn how the contractions are connected with other areas or functions of the body, such as respiration and other everyday activities.

• **Study the perineum and learn to appreciate both its localized and wider functions within the body.** The perineum occupies a small area, but has multiple and complex roles and interactions. There is a danger of focusing exclusively on it at the risk of creating unnecessary physical and psychological stress. It is important to continuously study its role within the body as a whole. For this reason, exercises for specific areas alternate with more global movements that engage the entire body.

• **Learn to recognize the psychological factors that arise during your study and exercise of the perineum.** The perineum is an area of formative body training and experience which can profoundly affect the psyche. Early sphincter training, sexual activity, and childbirth have psychological, emotional, social, and affective connotations. Thus many experiences associated with this area of the body are intensely marked by pleasure and/or pain, by relationships, by tenderness or negative judgements, and by acceptance and encouragement or rejection.

For some people, it is possible that certain exercises will provoke a resurgence of past experiences. Indeed, a period of companionship may be a good idea should such emotions prove too strong during the practice of certain exercises. While this is not the subject of this book, it is nonetheless an extremely important issue that is mentioned here and will be revisited during the practical exercises.

The pelvis

Form a clear mental image of your own pelvis

Most people have only a vague idea of the shape and volume of their own pelvis. It is often thought to be formed of small, smooth pieces. Yet a clear mental image of this bony belt is indispensable to precisely locating the movements and sensations that originate here.

Begin by reviewing the bony structures of the pelvis in Chapter 1, where it is described and drawn from many angles. Then, while looking at the drawings, try to *transpose them to your own pelvis.* The exercises in this book require that you be able to locate the:

- iliac crests
- pubic symphysis, the ischial tuberosities, and between them the ischiopubic ramus
- posterior superior iliac spines (PSIS, in the back at the top)
- sacroiliac articulations (lower down).

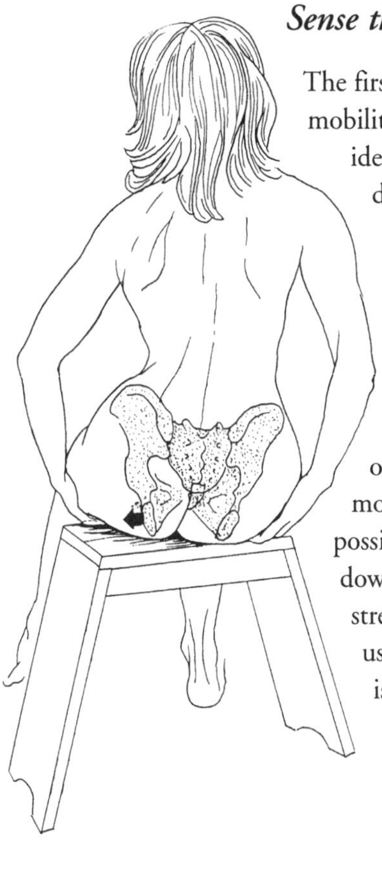

Sense the mobility of the pelvis

The first thing to discover here is the sensation associated with the mobility—however small—of the pelvic bones. To reinforce the idea that the pelvis is capable of very small changes in shape, do the following:

1. Lateral mobility

Sit down on a stool (the height of a normal chair) or on the ground, whichever you prefer, and lean on the ischial tuberosities. Lift yourself onto the right tuberosity, and take your weight off the left. Leaning into your hands, move the left ischium as far away as possible from the right. Then sit down, holding the two ischia stretched apart. (You can also use your hands to pull the ischia apart.)

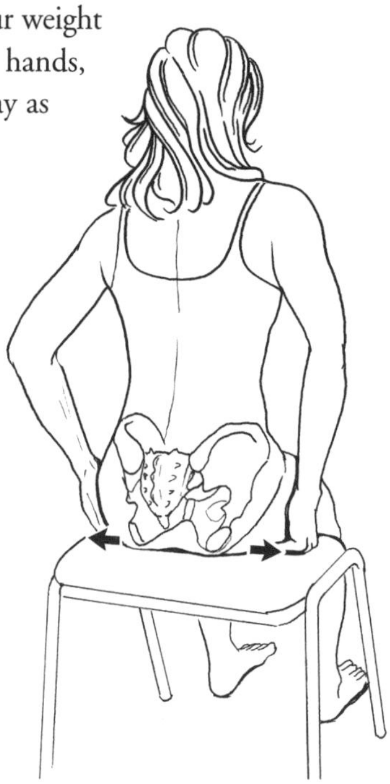

Do you now feel that you can have a wider base on your two ischia? Remain for a while in this position and take account of what it feels like.

Now move your weight onto the left tuberosity, raising the right tuberosity from the stool and bringing it as close as possible toward the left. Then put your weight back on the two tuberosities. Do you now feel that you can draw them together? Once again, identify the sensations, what it feels like. Repeat the same exercises on the left side. Try to find the full scope of movement through many repetitions on each side.

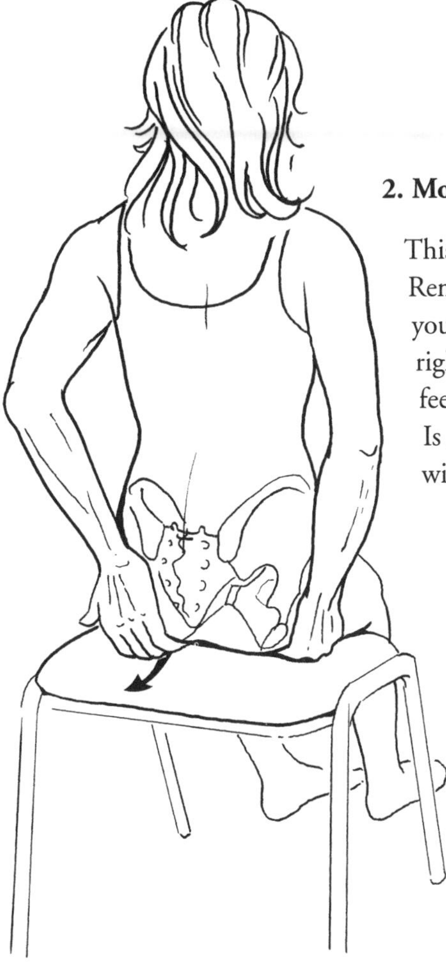

2. Mobility from front to back

This exercise is similar to the preceding one. Remain seated on the ischial tuberosities. Put your weight onto the left one. Now carry the right one as far forward as possible. Do you feel the asymmetry of the two tuberosities? Is it as though you have taken a step forward with one ischium? Once again, change sides.

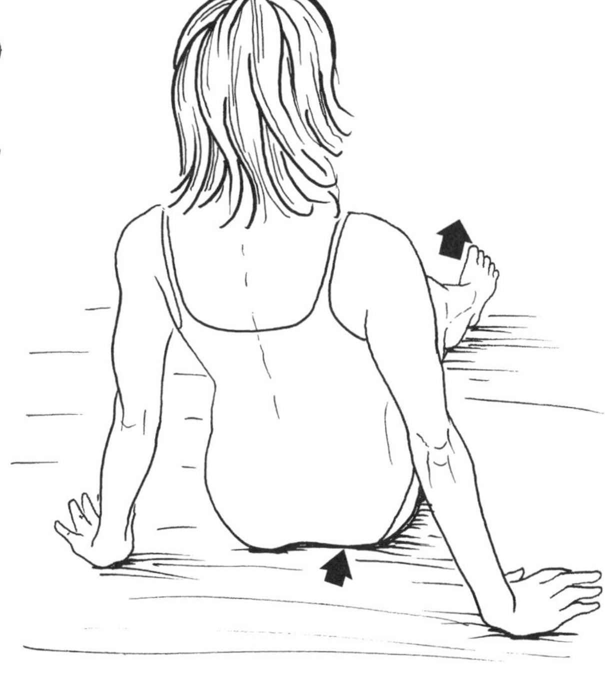

Rest for a moment in the starting position. Perhaps you will now notice that your usual sitting position is asymmetrical. This is quite common and contributes to the asymmetrical way we hold ourselves while standing.

Active mobilization of the pelvis

Sit on the ground with the knees open, leaning forward on your hands. (If that position is painful for your knees, sit on a chair, leaning forward on your hands in the same manner.) You should be able to lift the weight off your pelvis. Open the thighs a little so that the hips are free (unhindered by muscular tension from the thighs being held too wide) and the pelvis can move easily.

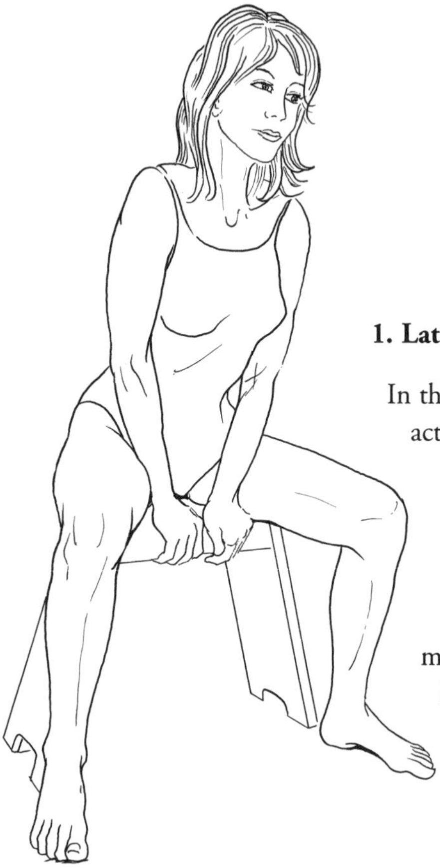

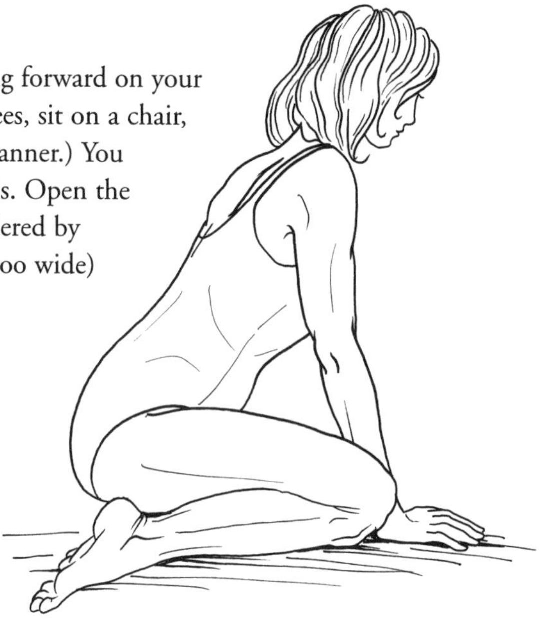

1. Lateral movements

In this position, repeat the previous movements, but more actively *try to spread the base of the pelvis between the two ischia.* To begin with, you can do this by an internal rotation of the thighs; however, this is not essential. The muscle that pulls your ischia apart in this case is the obturator internus.

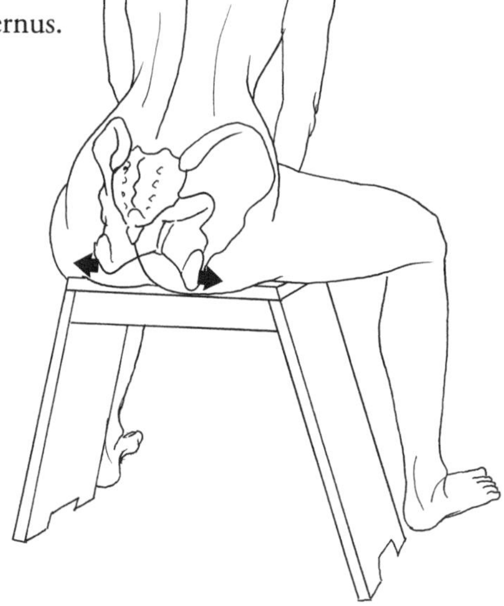

Now try to close the space between the two ischia. The muscles that bring them together are the gluteal muscles.

2. Front to back movements

Try and lift the coccyx up at the back as high as possible without arching the lumbar region and without rotating the pelvis in anteversion (forward tilting). The goal is to move only the sacrum and coccyx in the pelvis.

3. Combined mobilization

Now try to combine the movements of the three major bones. Spread apart the two ischia while at the same time lifting the coccyx. Imagine the iliac crests coming together at the top. The pelvis should feel completely open below at the level of the inferior opening.

Now do the opposite exercise: Bring the ischia together and pull the coccyx toward the pubis. Imagine the iliac crests opening at the top. The pelvis should feel considerably reduced in size at the bottom.

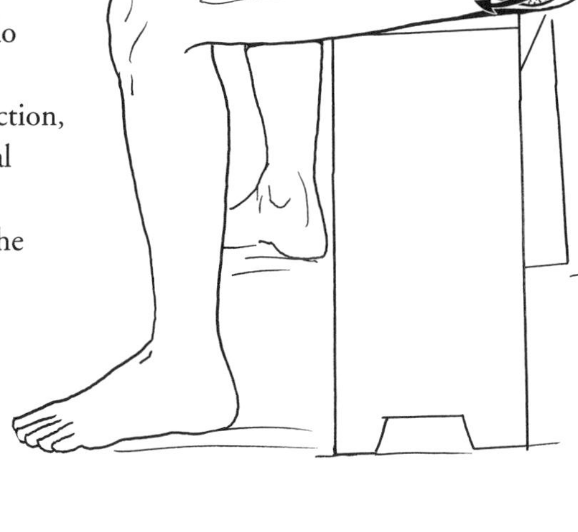

How to practice these exercises

- Alternate the movements between opening and closing a dozen or so times.
- Do not force the movements, but try to do them as fully as possible.
- When you finish a movement in one direction, let the pelvis return passively to its original position.
- Finally, breathe deeply before beginning the exercise on the other side.

All of these movements, even the smallest one, modify the shape of the lower pelvis and mobilize the joints, muscles, and internal organs. They *activate* the blood and lymphatic circulation in the whole area. Because of this, they are an excellent way to keep the lower pelvis healthy.

Use hip movements to mobilize the pelvis

1. Sitting: lateral mobilization

Sit on the ground, leaning back on your hands. Gradually open one thigh. In the beginning, try to do this movement in the hip joint only, without moving the pelvis. At a certain point (the "outer limit") the thigh cannot move out any further without drawing the pelvis with it toward the opened-out thigh.

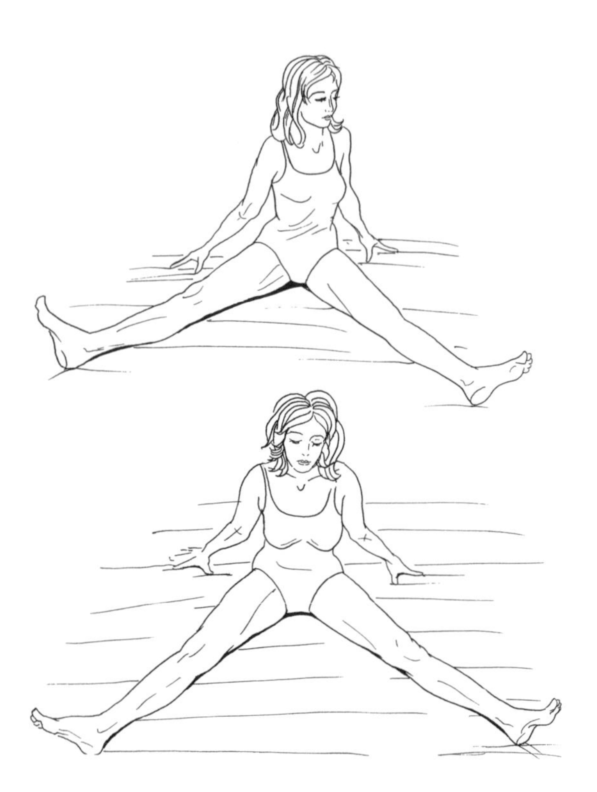

Go back to the initial position. Now do the same movement with both thighs, i.e., open them on the left and right sides at the same time. When you reach your outer limit, the pelvis no longer follows the thigh, but stays in place. However, pulled by the thigh muscles, it becomes slightly distorted. The pubis is pulled a little to the front, while the sacroiliac bones are compressed at the back.

2. Lying down: lateral mobilization

Repeat the same procedures lying on your back. Spread open one thigh. When you reach your outer limit, feel how the pelvis follows now: it leans to one side. Repeat again with both thighs. Do you feel how the pelvis "distorts" itself now? It's the lower parts of the pubic symphysis and the sacro-iliac joints that are stretched, while their upper limits are compressed.

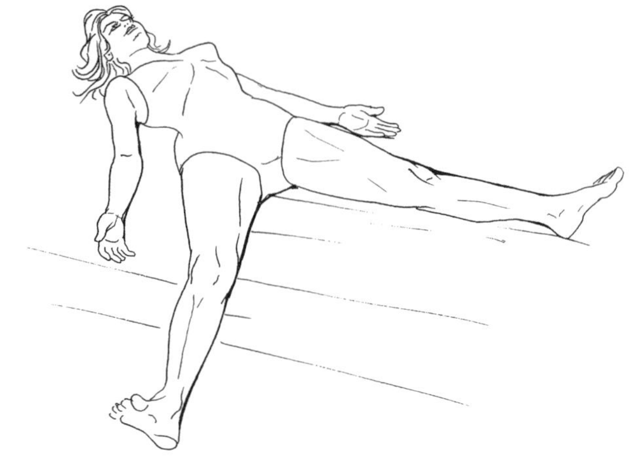

3. Lying down: mobilization from front to back

Lie down on your back, spreading out your arms on the floor, both to the same level. With your palms facing upward, use your hands to press against the floor to stabilize the thorax. Cross the right leg as far as you can over the left, crossing not only the leg but the thigh as well, by rolling the pelvis with it toward the left. Your shoulders, however, should stay on the floor. Flex the right knee and let it touch the ground without using force. Do you feel now that your pelvis is compressed in front, at the level of the pubic symphysis, rather than behind, at the level of the sacroiliac joints?

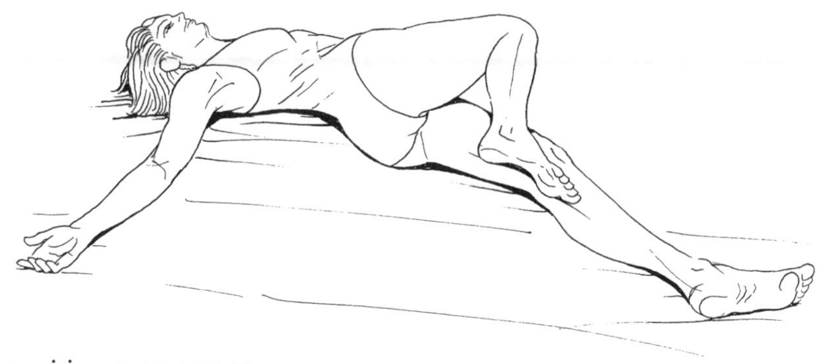

From this position, turn over to the left side. Now try to stretch your left leg as far as you can behind you while going as far as you can in front with the right leg. At the same time, try and straighten the right knee. (If you can get hold of the right foot in your left hand, you can hold on to it to help stretch out your knee.)

In this position, the two ilium bones are pulled in opposite ways. The right ilium is rotated posteriorly (pulled by the hamstrings), and the left ilium, conversely, is rotated anteriorly (pulled by the anterior ligaments of the left hip). The pubic symphysis is twisted and the sacroiliac bones are rotated.

From these few examples you can see that, nearly always, when you mobilize the hips, you slightly mobilize the pelvic bones between them. It is useful to practice these movements and many others in order to take care of the pelvic joints. This, in turn, will improve your sensory perception when you exercise the muscular structures.

Keeping the pelvis stable during hip movements

In a very different way, while practicing the previous exercises, you can *try to keep the pelvic bones from moving between themselves.* For example, in the first exercise, when you open the thighs, you can *try not to let the symphysis open,* but instead keep it pulled together as tightly as possible toward the front. In the same way, *try not to let the sacroiliac joints compress at the back,* but keep them as open (disengaged) as possible.

The exercises are then no longer done just to increase mobility. Rather, the aim is to encourage active involvement of certain muscles to keep the pelvis stable (these muscles will not be detailed here).

Mobilization of the pelvis on the hips: anterior and posterior rotation

1. Pelvic and then lumbar movements

- Get down on all fours.
- Rotate the pelvis as if you wanted to raise the coccyx or the ischia.

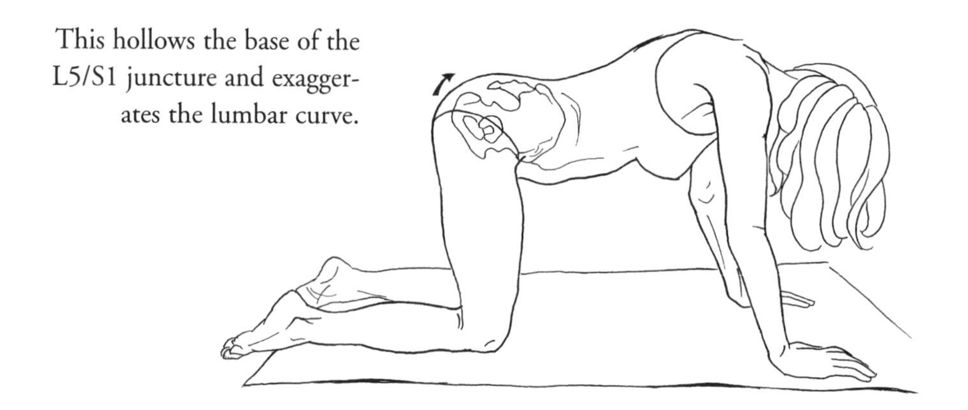

This hollows the base of the L5/S1 juncture and exaggerates the lumbar curve.

- Rotate in the opposite direction as if trying to tuck in your coccyx.
- Pull the ischia forward between the thighs.

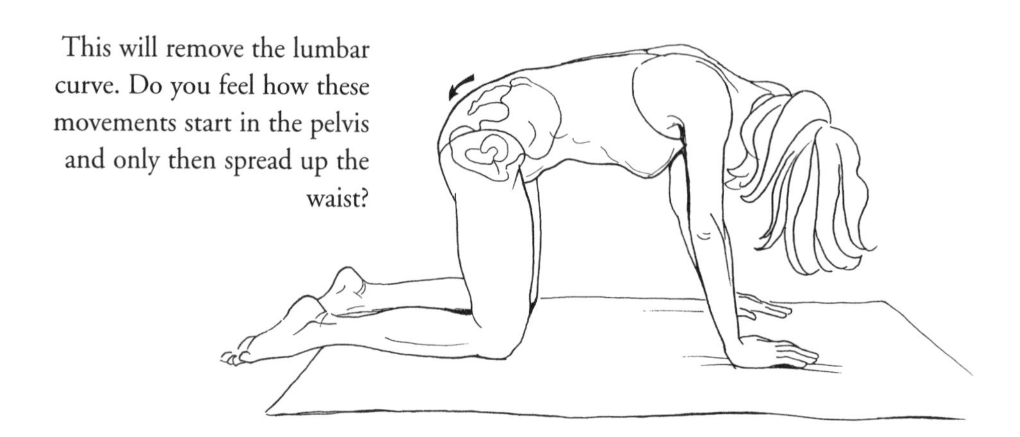

This will remove the lumbar curve. Do you feel how these movements start in the pelvis and only then spread up the waist?

2. Lumbar and then pelvic movements

Start in the same position as the previous exercise, and hollow the back, thereby *increasing the already existing curvature in the lumbar region.* Go as far as you can. Do you feel how this movement pulls the pelvis, if you let it, into anterior rotation?

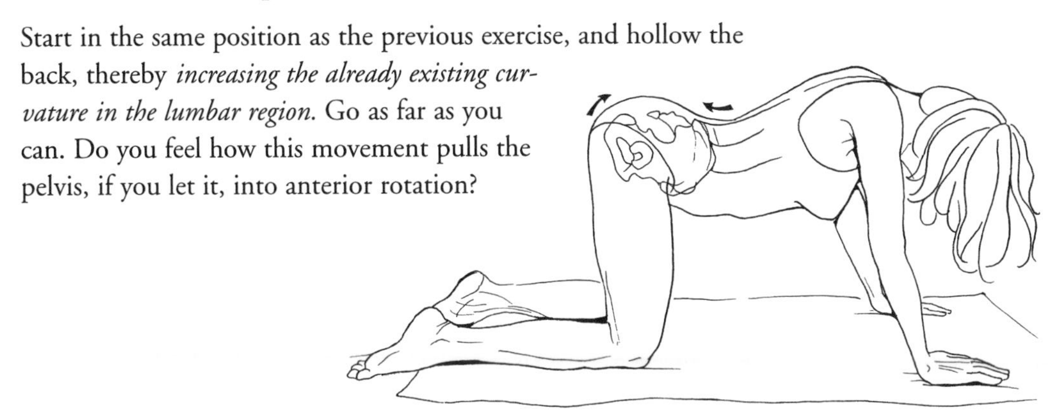

Now do the opposite. Try to pull the lumbar vertebrae into a *curve that rounds the back.* In doing this, one often only rounds the dorsal region. Do you feel how the movement involves the pelvis, drawing it into posterior rotation from the waist level? You can repeat this exercise a dozen or so times, beginning with movement of either the pelvis or the spine. In addition, you can synchronize your breathing with the exercises.

At the conclusion of the exercise session, it is a good idea to stretch out your back. Sit back on your heels and then lean forward, stretching out your hands on the ground as far away from you as possible. Do this during a good exhalation, keeping the position while breathing out deeply.

The muscles of the pelvic floor

First of all, you need to get to know this muscular area of your body. The following exercises will help you gain an awareness of the different muscles brought into play:

- those that respond to the pelvic floor under pressure
- those that make contact with the pelvic floor.

You will find that these exercises help you form a mental image of the two distinct muscular layers so that you can call on them and reinforce them separately.

Locating the pelvic floor muscles

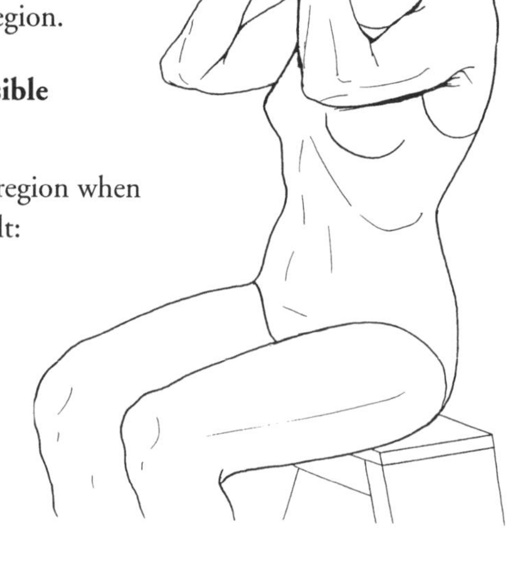

1. Feeling the pelvic floor muscles under pressure

In a sitting position, blow strongly into a balloon or mime the same action. You will immediately feel a region in the lower pelvis that comes into play as you blow. This, globally speaking, is the pelvic floor region.

2. Feeling and testing three different possible "responses"

Observe what happened in the pelvic floor region when you blew into the balloon. You may have felt:

- that the act of blowing into the balloon caused the *urge to urinate*
- that the pelvic floor was being *pushed downward*
- or, conversely, that the region was *contracting strongly in on itself* and even moving upward.

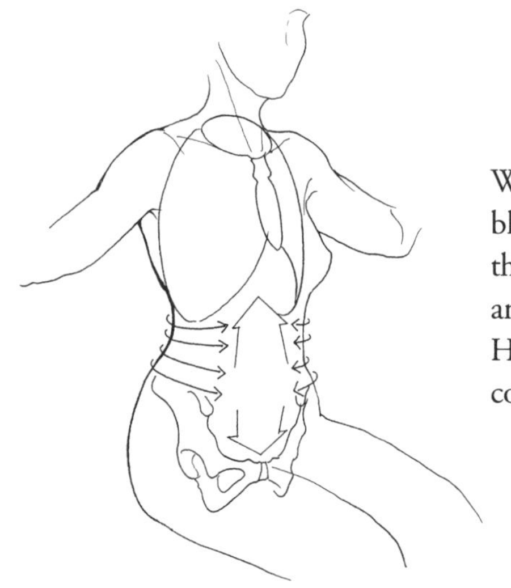

What is happening? To inflate a balloon, you have to blow air in under pressure. To create this high pressure, the abdominal muscles contract, pulling in the abdomen and pushing it, in part, upward and toward the thorax. However, part of the pressure moves downward, and compresses not the thorax but the perineum (see p. 76).

If the pelvic floor has *weak muscular tone,* this pressure will be enough to bring on an urge to urinate. If the pelvic floor muscles have sufficient tone, they will be able to control the urination, in which case you may simply feel the muscles contract more or less downward.

Alternatively, if the pelvic floor muscles have *strong tone,* they will play a different role: they will join the abdominal muscles in creating pressure that moves upward to the thorax. This is more unusual at the beginning. However, after you have practiced the exercises proposed in the following pages, together with those to synchronize the pelvic floor muscles with the abdominal muscles (see p. 118), you will gradually attain this level of muscular tone.

Thus, there are three possible responses to doing this exercise. Each one is dependent to varying degrees upon the muscular strength of the perineum and the extent to which the perineum can be "commanded" to contract at any given moment. This awareness is fundamental to precisely localizing the area to be exercised, and to distinguishing between the pelvic floor muscles and the adjacent muscles that are often confused with those of the perineum (see Chapter 4).

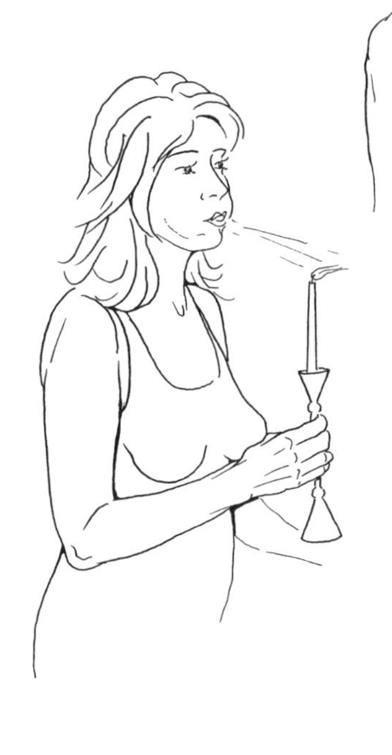

3. Try to notice the same sensations in everyday life

For example, when you:

- cough, feel the moment just before your cough
- raise your voice
- laugh
- block your breath before exerting yourself, as if lifting a heavy object
- blow out a candle flame.

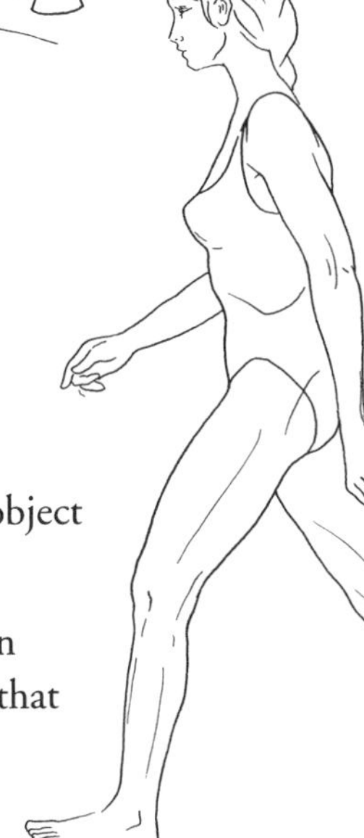

In all these situations the perineum is put under pressure. You can easily recognize the situations described above. Now you can see that the perineal muscles can be trained not only by practicing a series of exercises, but also by doing ordinary movements during an ordinary day.

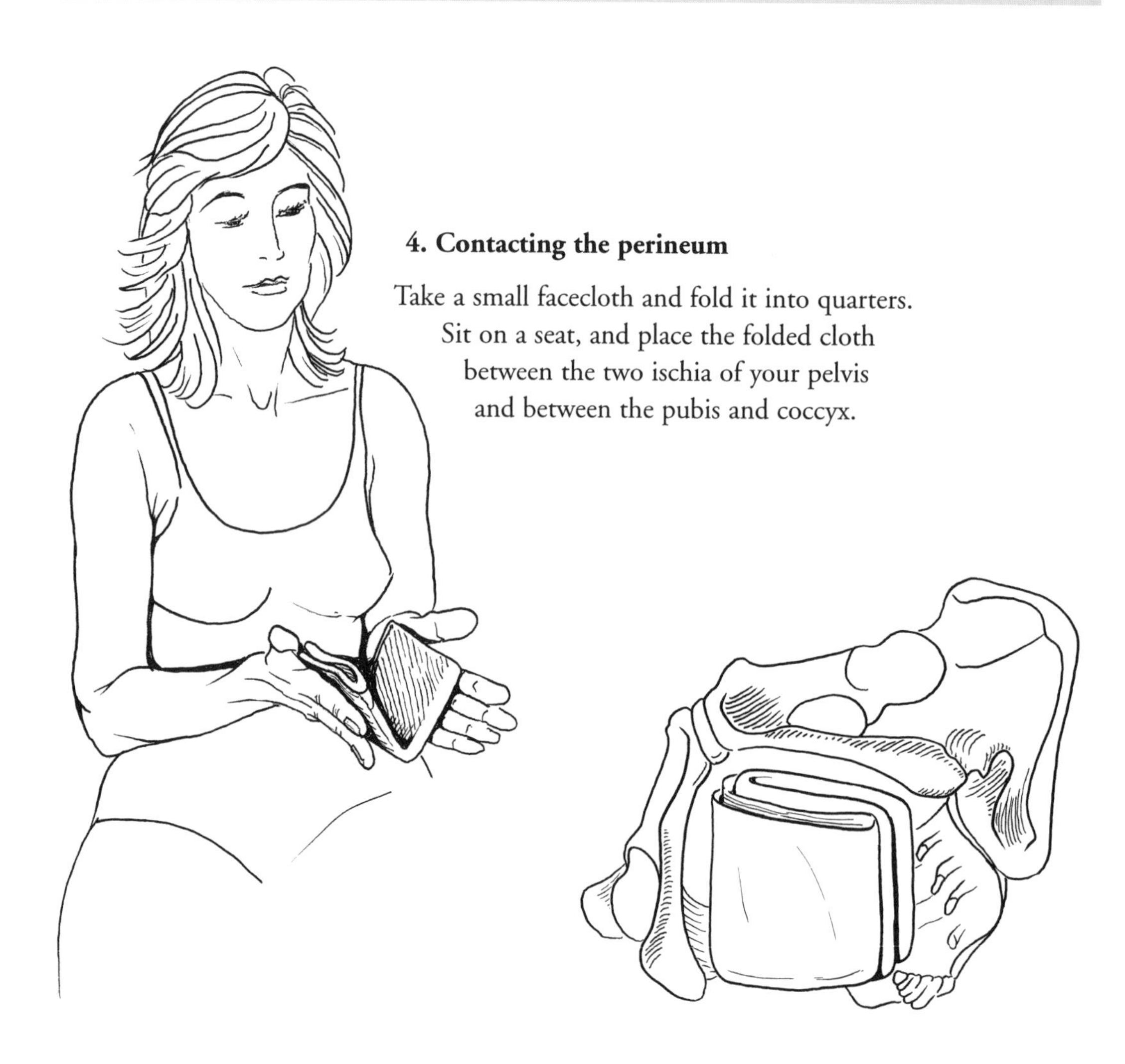

4. Contacting the perineum

Take a small facecloth and fold it into quarters. Sit on a seat, and place the folded cloth between the two ischia of your pelvis and between the pubis and coccyx.

What do you feel? Are you able to allow the region in contact with the facecloth to adapt itself comfortably? Do the following:

- Stay in this position, with the perineum in contact, and take a few deep breaths. Observe the different sensations while breathing in and breathing out.
- Using this contact, locate the three orifices and try to imagine the distance between each of them.
- Repeat the exercises from the preceding pages, i.e., blow into a balloon or mime the same action. Note that the region in contact with the folded facecloth overlaps the area put under pressure by the blowing action.
- Now take the folded cloth away. What do you feel? Does the region seem the same?

The exercises in this section enabled you to make two fundamental discoveries about your perineum:

1. You learned to *locate the region of the perineum* through exercises involving muscular contractions, placing the region under pressure and contact stimulus.
2. You developed an *awareness and apprecia-tion of the tone* of your perineal muscles.

Exercises for pelvic floor response: from relaxation to tonicity

We will now begin exercises to locate and reinforce the pelvic floor muscles. It is important to keep in mind one working principle: You should be able to make this region either very supple and relaxed or very activated. During delivery, what is needed is a pelvic floor capable of being stretched to its maximum without tearing. In other words, the muscles need to have an *elastic quality.* This elasticity is also necessary in more everyday situations, e.g., defecation, but also for respiration (see pp. 70-72).

On the other hand, after the delivery what is needed is a pelvic floor that is capable of actively supporting the lower abdomen and avoiding incontinence of the rectum and/or bladder. For this, the principal quality needed is *muscular tonicity.* This, too, is just as necessary for respiration.

Note: Elasticity and tonicity are not incompatible. They can, and even should, coexist quite comfortably. It is important to understand that reinforcing the muscular tonicity of the perineum will not compromise its suppleness and ability to stretch during the delivery. Similarly, exercises to relax and stretch this region will not interfere with reinforcing the same muscles. That having been said, some problems do occur in extreme cases, for example:

- Reinforcing an over-stretched perineum that contains a prolapse could be difficult and may require physical therapy.

- Attempting to relax a very muscular perineum (in athletic bodies) may also prove to be difficult. This could create an obstacle for the baby on the day of delivery.

Exercises to reinforce muscle tone will increase muscular strength, the tissues' vascularization, and thus its nutritional state. On the other hand, exercises that *only* reinforce muscle tone risk the formation of rigid and hypertonic muscles, which can mask the relatively subtle sensations associated with childbirth.

Exercises that relax and stretch the muscles will increase their elasticity and the mother's awareness of subtle and exact sensations. These exercises also contribute to increased muscular vascularization and nutritional state. The following pages will constantly repeat the importance of exercising both objectives simultaneously.

Contracting and strengthening the superficial muscles of the pelvic floor

These exercises mainly concern the superficial muscles of the pelvic floor (described on p. 36). Other muscles will be strengthened as well, especially when you first begin doing these exercises, as it is practically impossible to dissociate them.

1. Forming a mental image of the inferior opening

All four bony insertions of the superficial layer—the lower end of the pubic bone, the two ischia, and the coccyx—are easy to locate, as they are all externally palpable. *Note:* It is not unusual to imagine one's own ischia as being much further back than they really are. Take the time to look at the description of these four landmarks (pp. 14-24). If necessary, transpose them onto yourself.

You are lying on the circumference of the inferior opening, and the muscles you are about to contract are attached to the internal surfaces of the pelvic bones that form the opening. *Note:* When you are in an upright position, looking at your body from above, the inferior opening is below the deeper muscular layer.

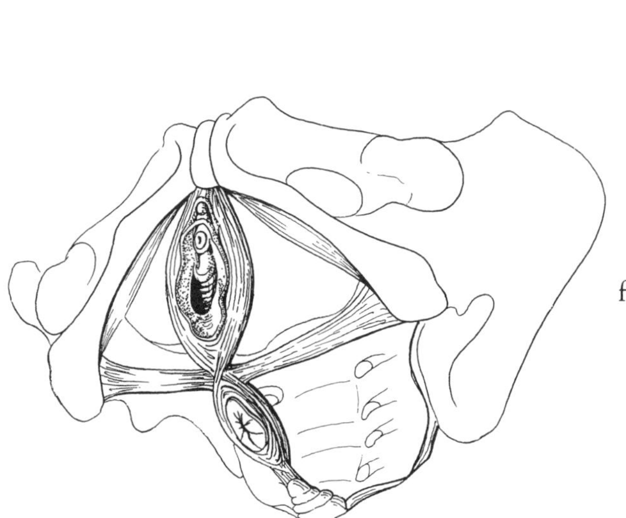

Now visualize the structure of the superficial muscular layer (see pp. 36 and 37), noting that it crosses over and forms a figure 8 from the front to the back.

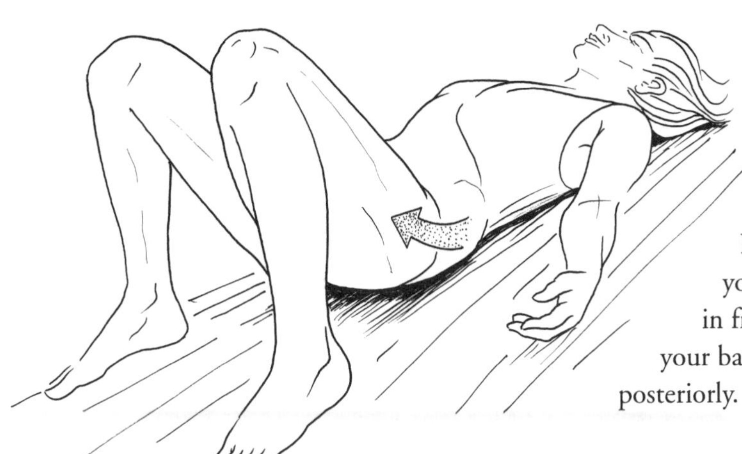

2. Contracting the muscles from front to back

Lie down on your back on a mat or mattress. Bend your knees, putting your feet flat on the ground in front of you. Now flatten your back, tilting the pelvis slightly posteriorly.

In this position, try to actively *draw your coccyx and pubis toward each other.* Relax, and then try repeatedly to identify the movement and the muscles. You are trying to feel a contraction along the median line (figure 8) of your perineum. Do not try to contract deep within the pelvis, nor should you look for a sensation of lifting. Rather, focus strictly on the back-to-front or front-to-back direction. You can check for the correct movement by placing a finger on the central tendon, or by placing your hand over the entire perineum. The movement and sensation you need to feel is just along the median line and close to the skin. Try to avoid contracting the sphincters.

The desired movement contracts the bulbospongiosus muscle, not the external anal sphincter muscles (see p. 36). In the beginning you will probably contract everything at once, the perineal muscles as well as the sphincters. You will become more accurate as you progress and repeat the exercise.

3. Contracting the muscles from side to side

Now try to make a muscular contraction as though you are *actively drawing your two ischial tuberosities toward each other.* The line of contraction is very different from that in the previous example. Here the muscles that are called upon run from side to side (the superficial transverse muscles). As before, try to feel a line running only along that one direction, and no longer from the front to the back. You can touch the area just inside the ischium to feel the contraction.

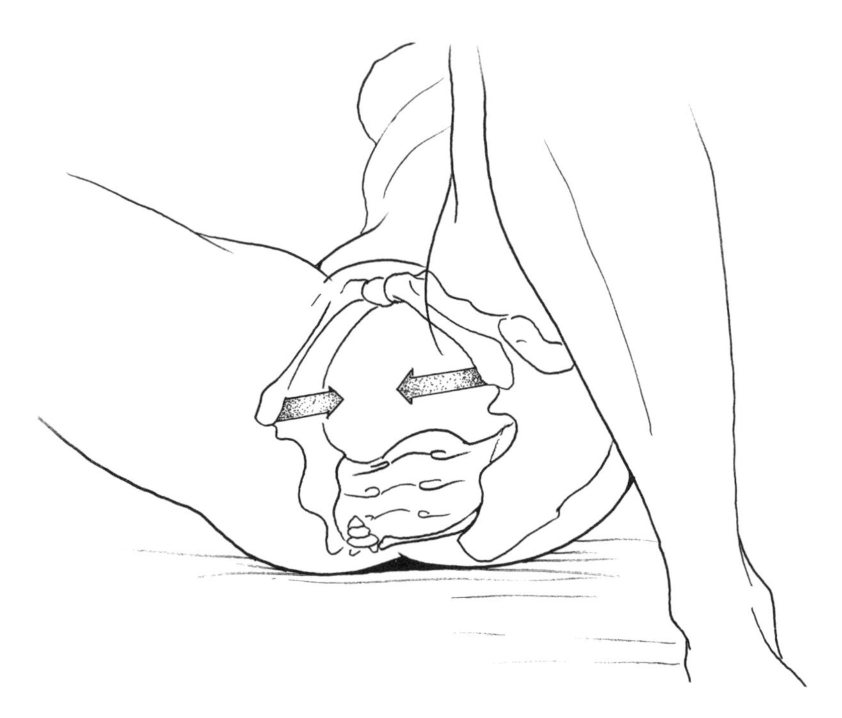

4. Varying the type of contractions

When you have found both lines of contraction, try to find them one at a time using the following progression:

- *A long contraction.* Hold the contraction for a few seconds (seven seconds is a good length of time) and then let go and relax for twice as long. Breathe deeply while you relax. Repeat the exercise five times.
- *Strong, quick contractions.* Now contract the muscles as strongly as you can. Keep them contracted for no more than two seconds. Then relax them completely and take a deep breath. Take care to work along the line from side to side. Repeat the exercise five times.

After contracting a muscle, remember to relax it completely. This moment of relaxation is very important:

- to avoid too much tension in your perineum
- to help you accurately recognize the muscular movements with more precision.

You need to be able to clearly distinguish the two muscular lines before beginning the next exercise, and this may take a few days of practice.

5. Crossed contractions

While still lying down, try to contract the two lines simultaneously. This may give rise to a sensation of pulling together the two lines of a cross drawn across the base of your perineum. *Note:* Unlike the contractions of muscles in the deeper layer, the contraction of the pelvic floor muscles is flat, and not a "lifting" contraction.

Follow this by repeating the process described on the previous page. Try to do longer contractions (for seven seconds), and try to make them as strenuous as possible (for only two seconds).

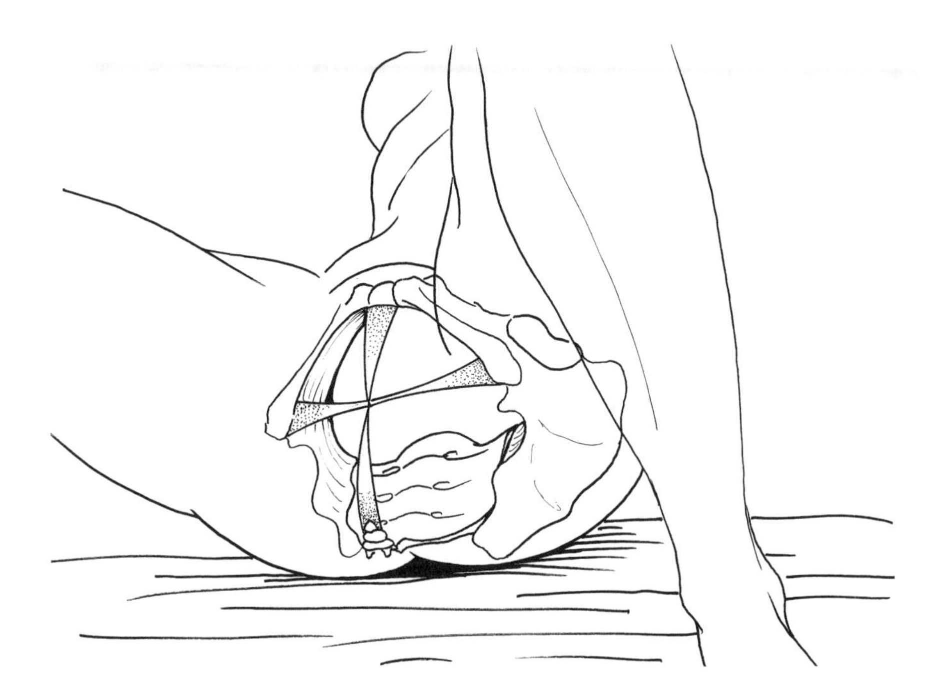

6. Coordinating the contractions with your breathing

During a long exhalation of about 15 seconds, as though you are gently saying "SSSSSSSS," contract the muscles. Now try doing the same thing with the letter "FFFFFFFF," letting your breath come out a little faster, and then with the sound "HHHHHHHH." For the latter, your breath will come out even faster. Feel yourself pushing out the last bit of air in the exhalations. Finally, you can try doing the contractions while laughing, coughing, jumping, or preparing to jump.

These exercises will allow you to coordinate muscular contractions of the superficial perineal layer with ordinary everyday breathing patterns. At the beginning, you will do this while exercising. Then you will begin to notice that you do it automatically whenever necessary. The contractions begin to become integrated into your body's reflexes.

You should also try to exercise regularly in order to maintain a level of tonus in these muscles, which are not often utilized in our sedentary lives. Always remember the principle: After an intense contraction, always allow for a relaxation of equal length.

Contracting and strengthening the deep muscles of the pelvic floor

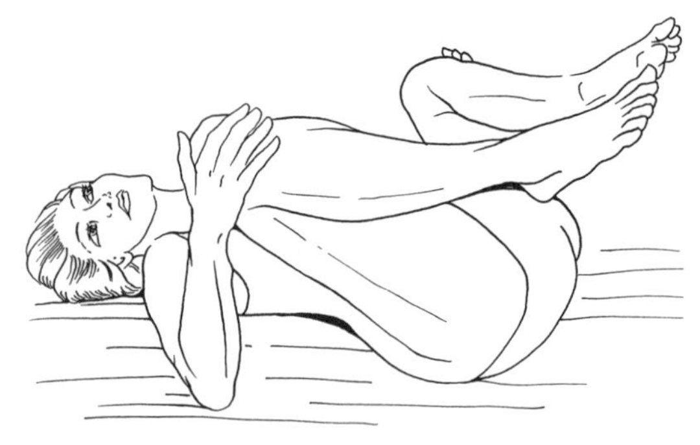

These exercises mainly concern the muscles that are attached to the middle opening (see pp. 22 and 39).

1. Forming a mental image

For a gentle exercise, lie down on your back or side with your knees drawn up toward your chest. For a more intense exercise, sit down with the ischia stretched apart, and for an even more intense workout, squat on your haunches.

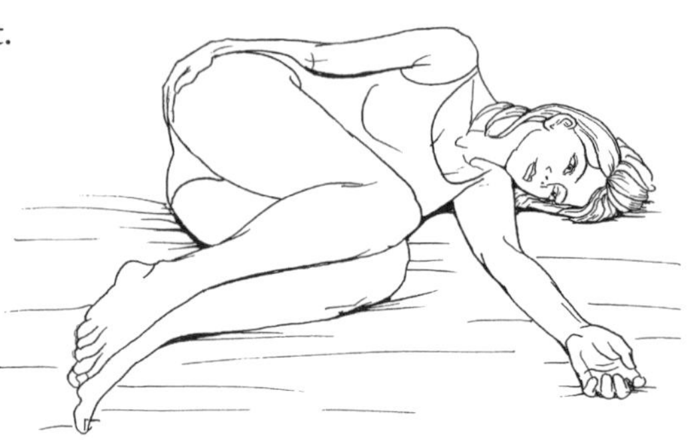

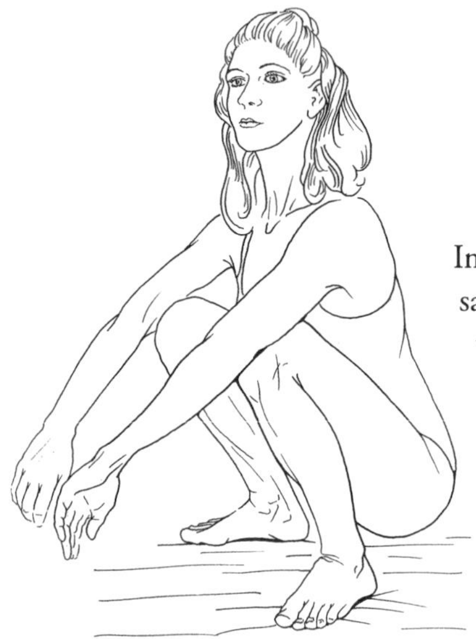

In this position, try to visualize your two ischia, the sacrum, and the pubic symphysis. *Mentally move upward* within the pelvis. You are no longer "skin deep." Rather, you are higher by five centimeters (two inches), at the level of the middle opening.

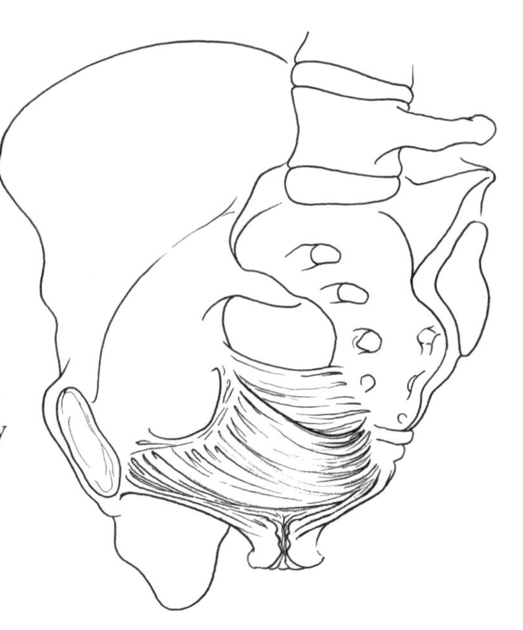

2. Contracting the whole deeper layer

Try to draw the muscles upward and inward. The *contraction pulls the anus upward* and may cause it to come forward as well. However, try not to confuse this movement with the previous ones. Just try to draw the muscles upward and inward.

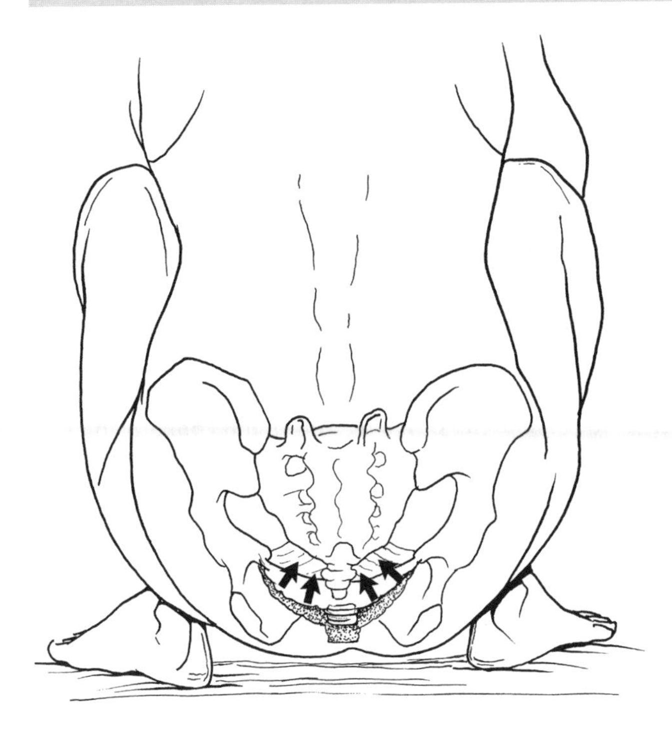

Here are some suggestions to help you locate the deeper layer:

- Try not to contract the anal sphincter, but rather just draw the anus itself upward. Contracting the anal sphincter generates a very different feeling from the one needed here. If necessary, refer to the exercises for the anal sphincter (p. 134).
- Try to get the sense that this is a contraction of a muscular "cloth" that stretches across the entire basin and pulls the vagina and the urethra with it. It is not a contraction in the middle that you are looking for, but a larger one using the muscular fibers along the outer reaches of the "cloth," inside the margins of the lower pelvis.

Then relax as completely as possible, breathing and trying to feel the weight of the internal organs dilating the area you just contracted.

Keep in mind the two key sensations that you have practiced with thus far: the *surface contractions* and the *drawing-upward contraction.* Repeat the same exercise a few times, contracting and relaxing this entire area to familiarize yourself with the sensations that are generated. Note the difference between the sensations in the present exercise and those of the previous exercise, which were tied to skin-deep muscular "lines."

3. Contracting the three layers of the pelvic floor upward

Try, as in the previous exercises, to exhale while making the consonant sound "FFFFFF," but this time bring the pelvic floor upward in stages, visualizing the three layers in the lower pelvis, like going "up the staircase":

- *First stage.* Pull up just a little, as far as the first surface layer. Sustain this for five seconds, trying to keep your breathing easy and regular. Now let go completely and breathe deeply.
- *Second stage.* Pull up a little further, as though you wanted to move into the next layer. Once again, hold it for a few seconds, and then relax by breathing deeply.
- *Third stage.* Pull up as high as possible, visualizing yourself moving up to the third layer. Try and pull up the entire surface of the pelvic floor, not just the sphincter. Relax for five seconds, maintaining a regular rhythm of breathing. Then relax completely. Once again, notice how the weight of the internal organs dilates the muscular region.

Repeat all three stages a few more times.

4. Contracting the three layers of the pelvic floor in a downward direction

You can also come "down the staircase" in stages. Recall that, as you went up, you contracted strongly. However, as you come back down, work a layer at a time, stopping a couple of seconds between each "floor." When you reach the final layer, relax completely and take several good deep breaths.

In the beginning, you will probably forget to breathe, i.e., you may block your breath. Now, however, after you have learned how to go up or come down in stages, try and coordinate your breathing in a fluid and regular fashion during the entire process of:

- going up
- staying at each layer, and
- going down toward the superficial layer.

5. Rapid contractions

Repeat the previous exercise, this time going up through all three layers at once by contracting strongly. Stay there for just a couple of seconds, then relax suddenly and completely for a few seconds. Breathe. Repeat this a few times. What makes this exercise different from the preceding one is that you contract and relax much faster. This will prepare you for moments when the pressure on the perineum suddenly increases, e.g., when you sneeze or cough.

6. Asymmetrical contractions

The deep layer of the pelvic floor is shaped like the inside of a bowl and contains the pelvic organs. It is quite possible to make it *contract only to the right or to the left,* leaving the other half relaxed. This will feel as though you are lifting only one side of the abdominal mass. It is not unusual, at the beginning, to contract other muscles at the same time, such as the cheek, jaws, hands, or feet. This, however, will gradually disappear.

7. In daily life

You can learn to integrate these exercises whenever your perineum is under pressure from everyday actions, such as sneezing, coughing, laughing, jumping, running, or carrying heavy objects (see p. 76).

Exercises for the puborectalis muscle

The most central part of the deep layer is the puborectalis muscle (see p. 39). It runs along the urogenital hiatus. As we have seen in Chapter 2, this is a vital passageway for childbirth. Yet it is also an area of potential weakness as the anterior perineal organs are not supported from beneath. The puborectalis muscle borders the three organs and creates a thick wall alongside this hiatus.

The strength of the puborectalis muscle is indispensable for supporting the internal organs, particularly the bladder and the uterus. And because it forms a sling around the orifices (especially the anus), the muscle also plays an important part in *voluntary continence* (see p. 61). Weakness in this muscle predisposes the individual to prolapse and incontinence. The following exercises are intended for strengthening this muscular bundle within the deep layer.

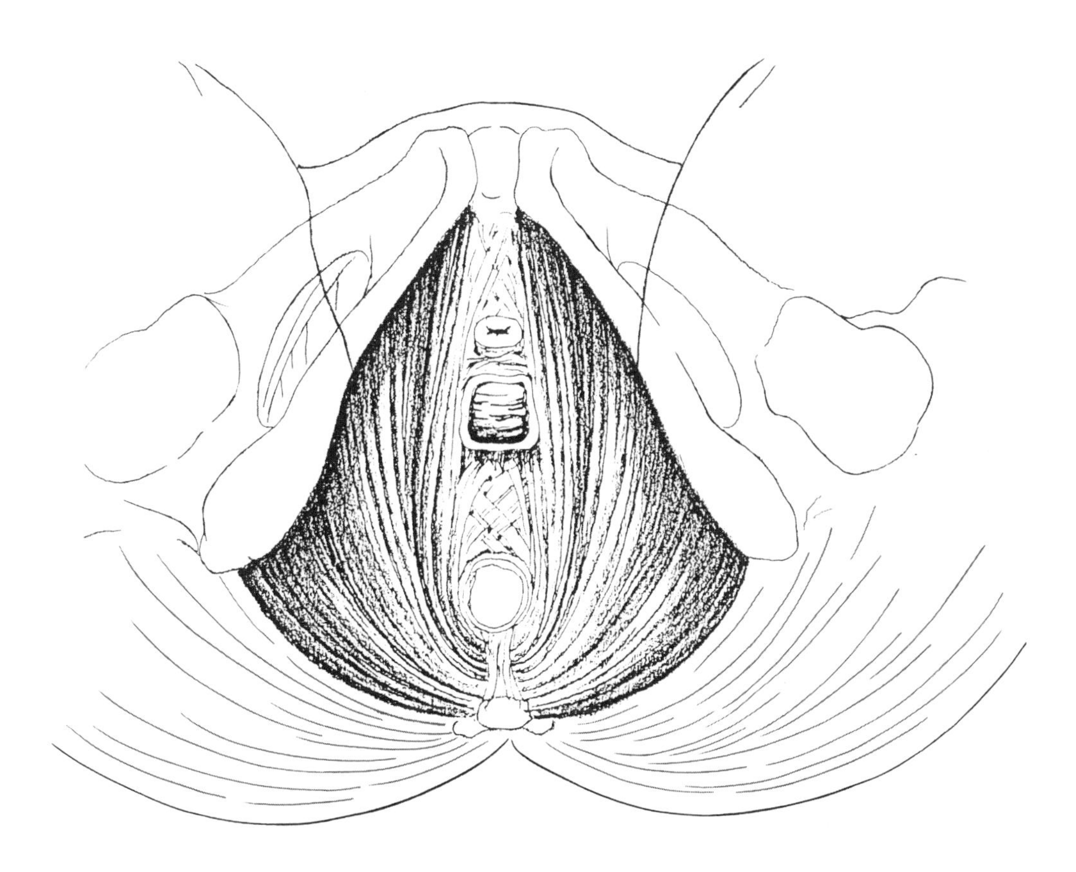

1. Forming a mental image of the puborectalis muscle

Begin by visualizing the three orifices along the median line of the perineum: the ureter, the vagina, and the anus. As with the preceding exercises, go up each of the passageways three or four centimeters above the median line. Now imagine, at this depth, that each passageway is surrounded on its left and right by a muscular girdle that begins at the pubis, runs along the sides of the three organs, then around the back of the anus, forming a long, narrow, U-shaped bundle. This muscular girdle is approximately two centimeters thick, more if in good tone.

2. Contracting the puborectalis muscle

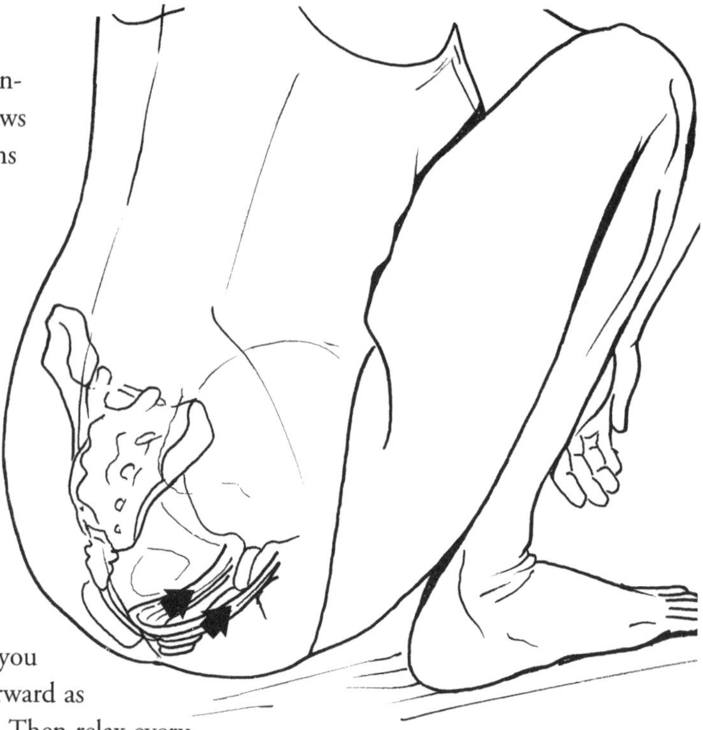

When this U-shaped muscle contracts, it does two things: It draws the anus forward, and it thickens to the left and right of the orifices.

Before you begin the exercises for the puborectalis bundle, repeat the overall contractions of the deep layer as seen on p. 138. Next, try to bring up the muscular hammock in its entirety, lifting it as a wide surface to a level high up in the pelvic cavity. Remain at this level, as though you were on a platform. While you are here, try to pull the anus forward as far as you can toward the pubis. Then relax everything, and breathe deeply. Repeat this double exercise a few times.

3. More intensive strengthening

You can now try to advance even further in three steps:

- Breathe out, pulling up the puborectalis bundle in its entirety. Stay there. Breathe in again. Breathe out once again, and pull the anus forward horizontally. Stay there. Breathe in without letting go of the contraction that pulls the anus forward.
- Breathe out again, and pull the anus forward a bit more. Stay there without letting go of this more intense contraction, then breathe in again.
- Breathe out and contract the muscle even more, until you feel as if you are moving the anus toward the pubis as much as possible. Then relax totally and breathe deeply.

Repeat this exercise two or three times, but more importantly, try to practice it over a number of consecutive days. You will soon notice that you are making progress in your ability to feel the different stages, and in the strength with which you are able to hold a contraction (which is not possible during the first few days). Later on you should try to practice this exercise regularly in your everyday life, perhaps once a day.

When you begin this exercise, you will find that it is practically impossible to avoid contracting the lower abdominal muscles. Once again, regular practice will help you make the necessary distinction.

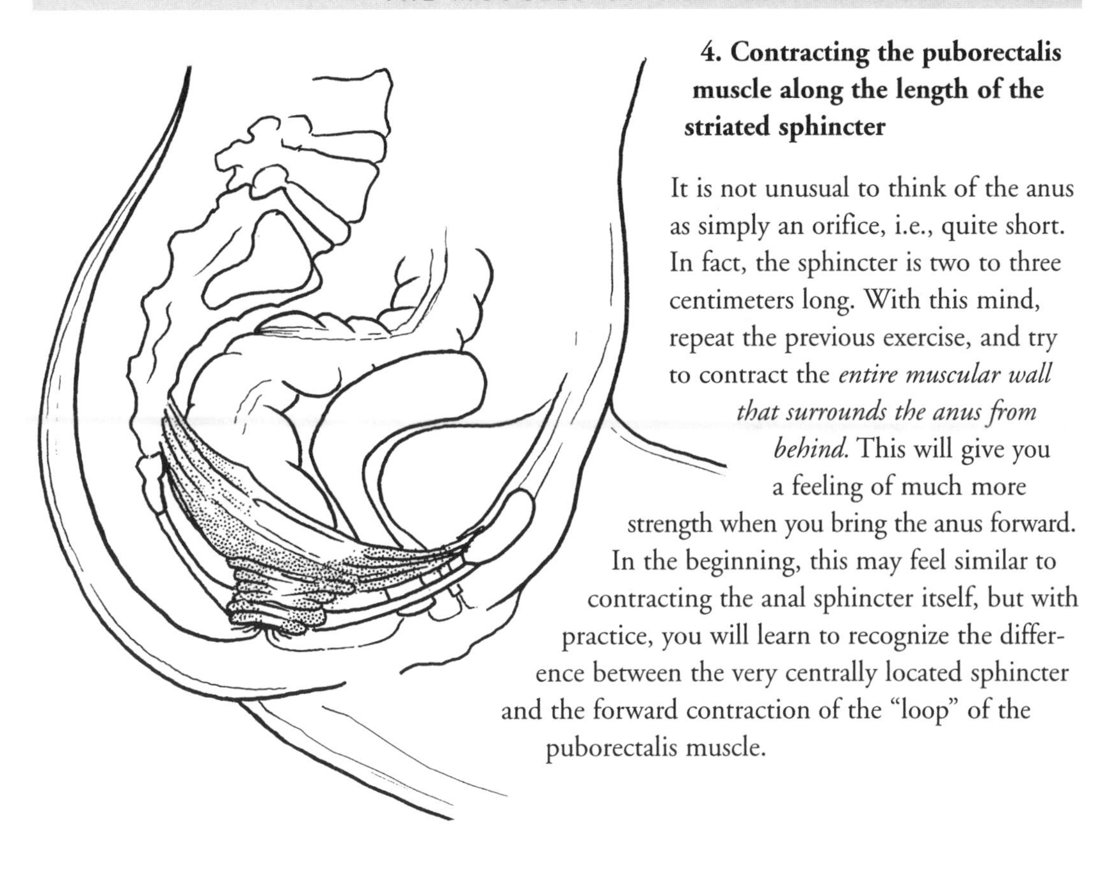

4. Contracting the puborectalis muscle along the length of the striated sphincter

It is not unusual to think of the anus as simply an orifice, i.e., quite short. In fact, the sphincter is two to three centimeters long. With this mind, repeat the previous exercise, and try to contract the *entire muscular wall that surrounds the anus from behind.* This will give you a feeling of much more strength when you bring the anus forward. In the beginning, this may feel similar to contracting the anal sphincter itself, but with practice, you will learn to recognize the difference between the very centrally located sphincter and the forward contraction of the "loop" of the puborectalis muscle.

5. Contracting the puborectalis muscle on one side only

The right and left muscles can be made to contract separately, like drawing on the reins of a horse. Repeat the second bulleted exercise from the previous page, but this time try to pull the anus forward using only the right muscle. Allow the left side to be as relaxed as possible. This creates a line of force that borders the ureter and vagina on the right side.

Here again, you can intensify this exercise by making the contractions in three stages, as described on p. 113. After completing the exercise on one side, breathe deeply and wait a while before doing the exercise on the other side.

Little by little, you will get to know the contractile response of each side, and its ability to sustain a long-held contraction. It is quite possible that you will find one side to be weaker than the other. You should then work to strengthen that side, and perhaps on certain days, exercise only that muscle. Working to find the contractions in these lateral muscles is an important step in the process of constructing a secure border to the urogenital hiatus.

6. More sustained exercises and integration with everyday life

You can now practice doing all of these exercises in different situations, some of which may increase the pressure on the perineum, such as blowing or coughing.

The muscles adjacent to the perineum

Exercises for the abdominal muscles

The exercises recommended here are not just concerned with strengthening the abdominal muscles. Rather, they are intended to coordinate with the exercises for the perineum. This will help avoid many problems that can occur at the level of the perineum, if ignored.

1. Feeling the abdominal muscles contract and the pelvic floor relax

This sequence is called an inverted perineal command, and this exercise is exactly what you should try to *avoid* during pregnancy and immediately after delivering the baby.

Lie down flat for the first exercise, knees bent, and feet flat on the floor. Allow the pelvic floor muscles to relax completely. Saying the consonant "SSSSSSSS" sound, breathe out completely, right down to your navel or waistline. This may take a few seconds.

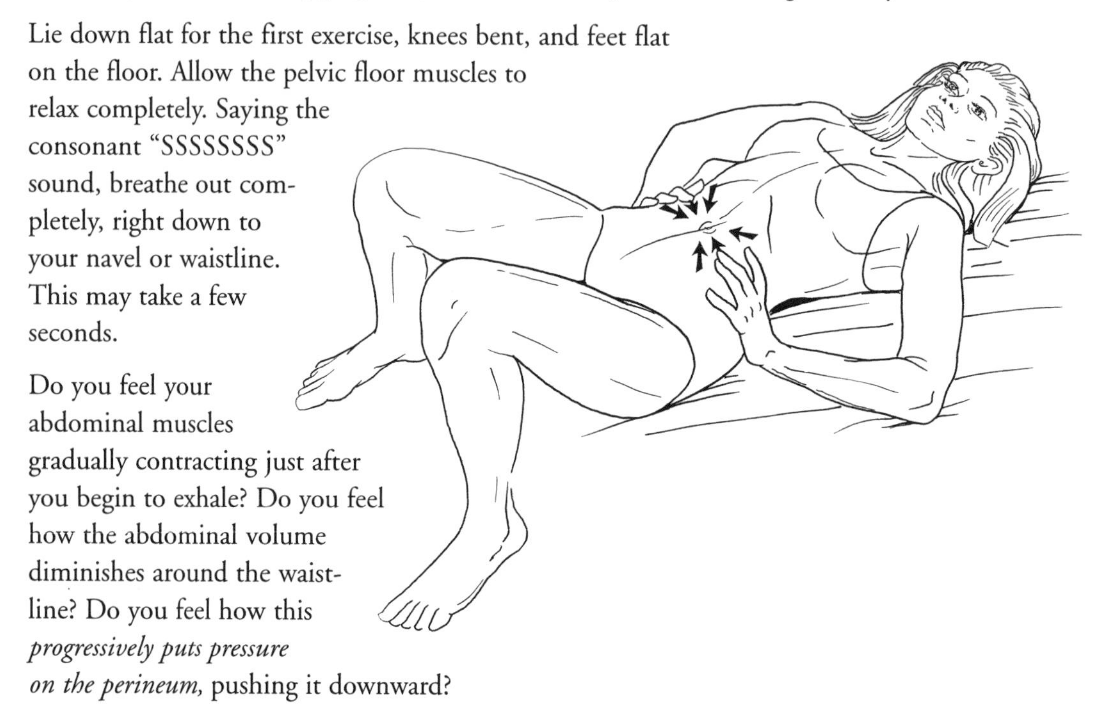

Do you feel your abdominal muscles gradually contracting just after you begin to exhale? Do you feel how the abdominal volume diminishes around the waistline? Do you feel how this *progressively puts pressure on the perineum,* pushing it downward?

This could be thought of as contributing to an "hourglass" musculature.

Do the same thing with the "FFFFFFFF" sound. Your exhalation should be faster and stronger. Then do the "HHHHHHH" sound; it should be more forceful. Finally, cough while doing the exercise. You should find that it is even quicker and stronger.

Repeat this exercise a few times so that you can really *feel* the following sequence of:

abdominal contraction → tightening around the middle → pressure on the perineum, which then descends if the pelvic floor is atonic.

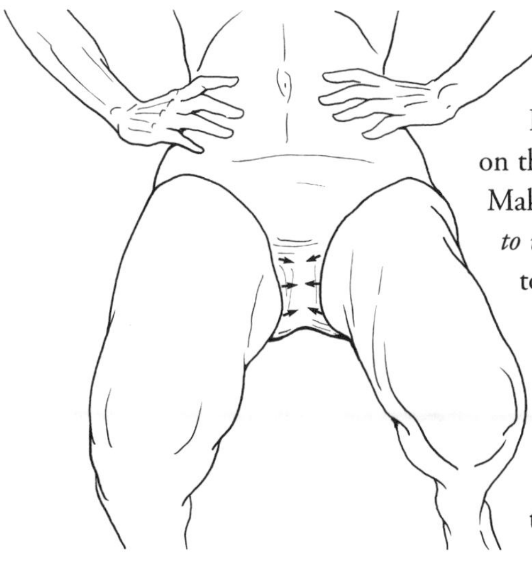

2. Feeling the pelvic floor contract and the abdominal muscles relax

Lie down on your back, knees bent, and feet flat on the floor. Now let the abdominal muscles relax. Make the "SSSSSSSS" sound as you exhale, and *try to visualize the breath starting at the perineum* (similar to the exercises on pp. 111 and 113). The exhalation begins with a contraction of the perineum. Then you will feel the abdominal muscles joining in. *Stop at that moment.* Breathe in again, and then start again. Repeat this a dozen or so times to help form a new habit, i.e., to contract the perineum during exhalation. Now repeat the process with the "FFFFFFFF" and "HHHHH HHH" sounds, and notice that the abdominal muscles are contracting sooner. Finally, do the exercise while coughing, which exerts the maximum force in the minimum time.

3. Synchronizing the pelvic floor muscles with the abdominal muscles

Be sure that you understand the previous exercises before beginning this one. To avoid any confusion, you should perhaps wait until the next day.

Lie down on your back, knees bent, and feet flat on the floor. Again, breathe out while making the "SSSSSSSS" sound, and *begin the contraction in the perineum.* Then, during the main part of the exhalation, *bring only the lowest abdominal muscles into play,* the muscles that would be covered by a bikini. When you feel the contraction reach the waist level, stop. *Breathe deeply, and relax fully after each contraction.* Reinforce this new movement using the "FFFFFFFF" and "HHHHHHH" sounds, and finally with a cough. Be careful not to relax the perineum when the abdominal muscles start to contract. To check your contractions, place two fingers on the central tendon, between the anus and the vulva, and the other hand on the lower abdomen.

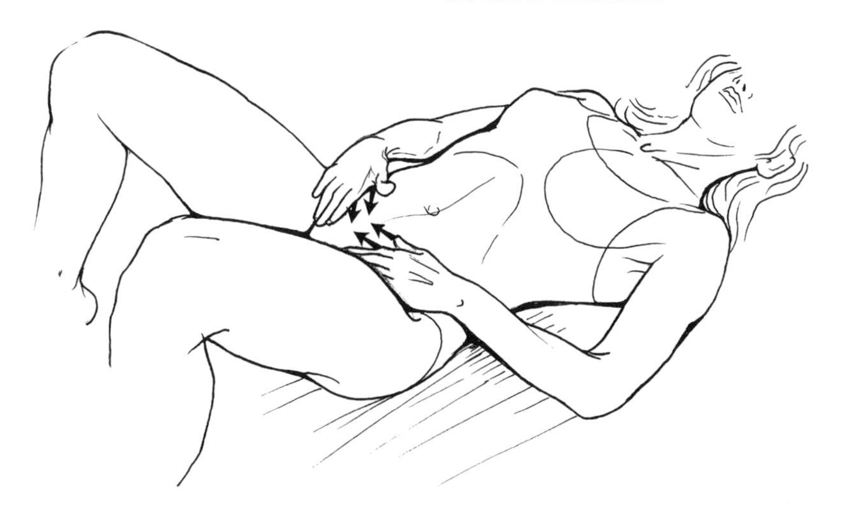

Synchronizing the movements of the pelvic floor muscles and the abdominal muscles is the key to caring for the perineal muscles. This should now become somewhat automatic for you. As with all conditioning, you need to repeat the exercise as many times as necessary. A good workout might be ten consecutive times, morning and evening, over a few days. This will, of course, depend on your own personal rhythm and exercise habits.

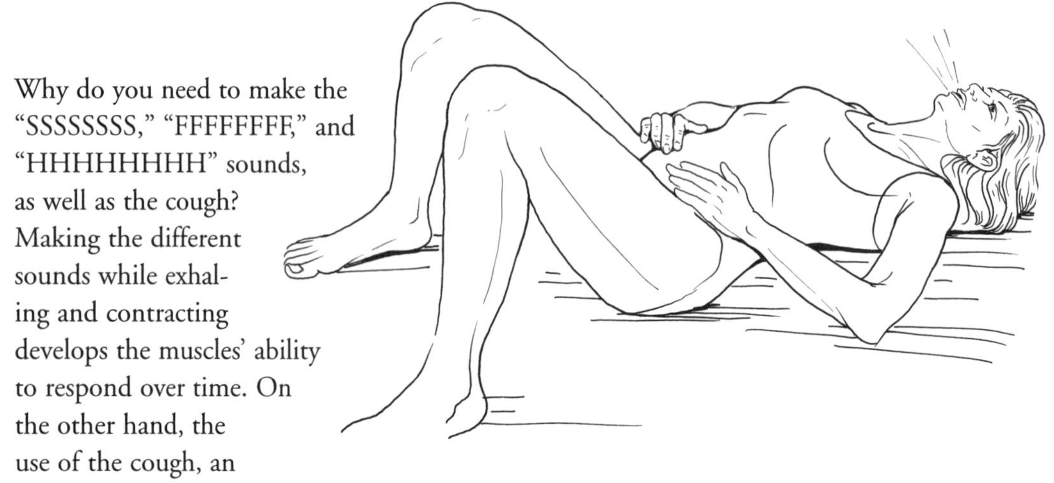

Why do you need to make the "SSSSSSSS," "FFFFFFFF," and "HHHHHHHH" sounds, as well as the cough? Making the different sounds while exhaling and contracting develops the muscles' ability to respond over time. On the other hand, the use of the cough, an intense and rapid contraction, prepares the muscles to respond to sudden strong demands such as sneezing, sudden bursts of laughter, or jumping.

4. You don't always need to coordinate the contraction with an exhalation

Lie down on your back, knees bent, and feet flat on the floor. Breathe out with the "SSSSSSSS" sound, and again, contract the pelvic floor, followed by the lower abdominal muscles. At the end of the exhalation, instead of relaxing, hold the contraction and breathe in again using the diaphragm, blowing up all but the lower part of the abdomen. Repeat as before, making the "FFFFFFFF" and "HHHHHHHH" sounds, as well as the cough.

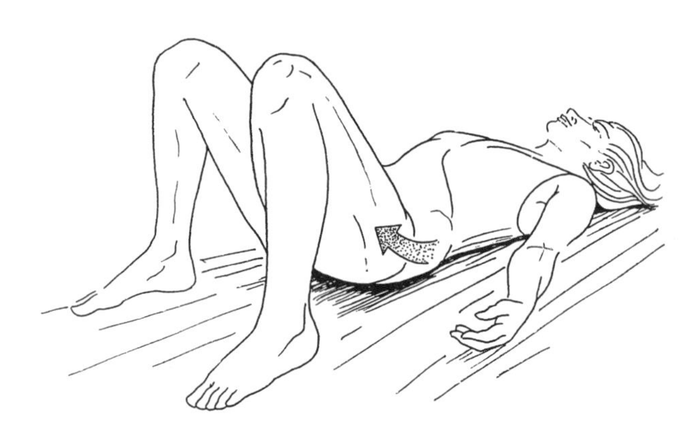

5. A more intensive exercise

When you are comfortable with the previous exercise, you can combine it with more intensive exercises for the abdominal muscles. Remember to relax and breathe deeply after each effort. Each of these exercises is performed lying down on your back, knees bent, and feet flat on the floor.

First, breathe out and roll the pelvis into retroversion, i.e., lift the coccyx off the ground.

Lift up your head, drawing your chin in toward the chest. Repeat the exercise, but this time pull your shoulders upward in the same movement. Repeat the exercise again, but this time make these motions while performing the first three exercises in this section (see pp. 118-119).

Flex your knees upward toward the chest.

Repeat the exercise, but this time place your hands on the knees and make a movement as though you were pushing them away, all the while keeping them drawn up. (Do not arch your back.)

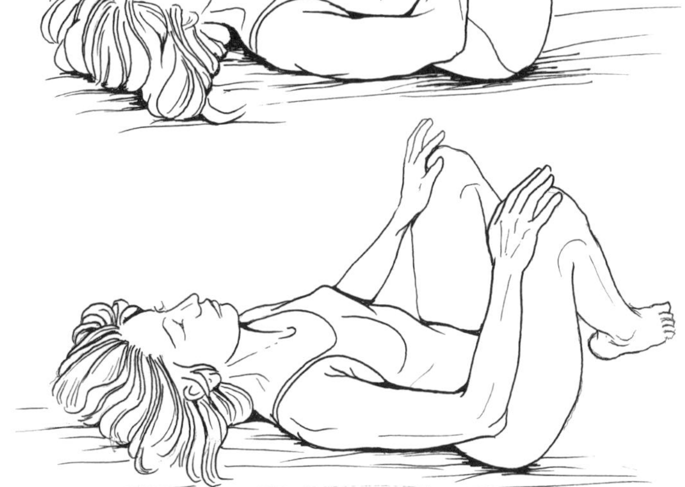

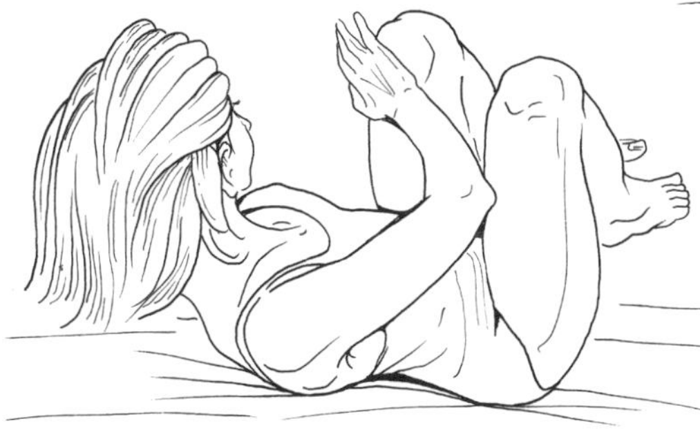

Repeat the previous exercise, but this time use your right hand to push away the left knee. Repeat the exercise again, but this time use your left hand to push away the right knee. Repeat with your head lifted or with the head and shoulders lifted.

6. Integrating these exercises into daily life

When, e.g., you:

- Get out of bed by lifting your trunk into the upright position. Make a habit of starting this movement from the pelvic floor.
- Basically repeat the previous exercise when you attempt to sit down or rise from a chair, or when you get in and out of a car. You can also do it when you lean forward with the upper body straight, or when you're carrying a heavy object.

Exercises for the gluteal muscles

1. Locating the contractions of the gluteal muscles

While lying down with your back on the floor, use a stool or other object of similar height to raise your feet. You may prefer to place a folded towel or cushion on the stool so that its edges do not hurt your ankles.

Keep your feet parallel to each other on top of the stool as you lie on your back. Spread out your arms. Now try lifting your back in a straight line with your legs so that your weight rests only on your shoulder blades and on the stool. To help achieve this, *raise the pelvis as high as possible.*

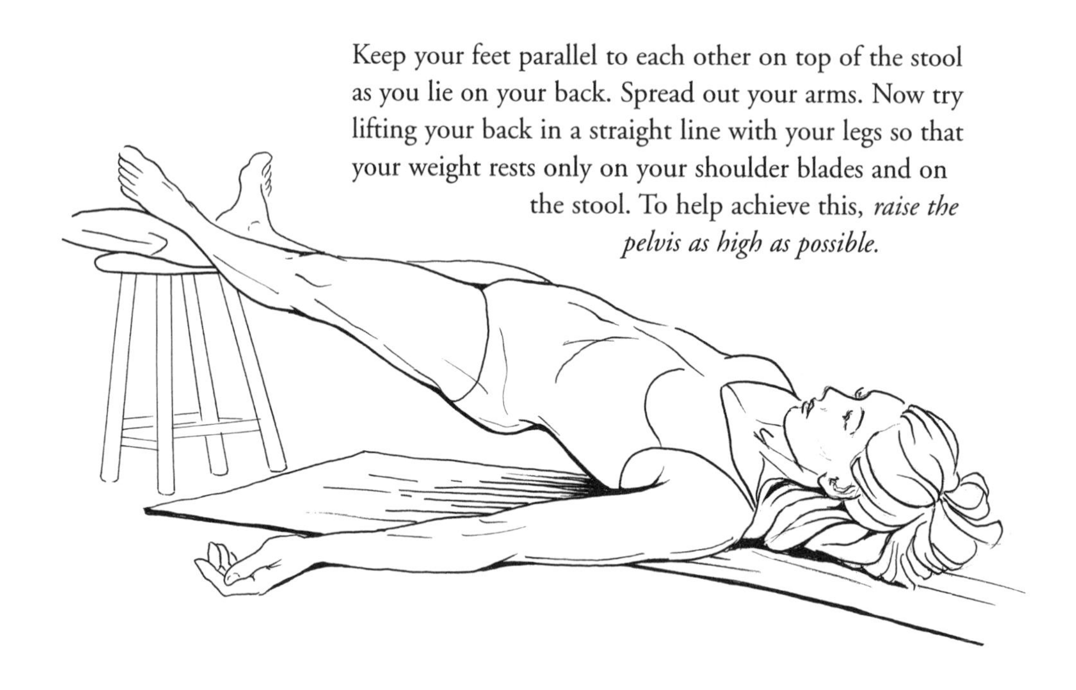

Now try to lift the pelvis into *posterior rotation,* i.e., move as though you were lifting yourself up by the coccyx. Do you feel the gluteal muscles contracting?

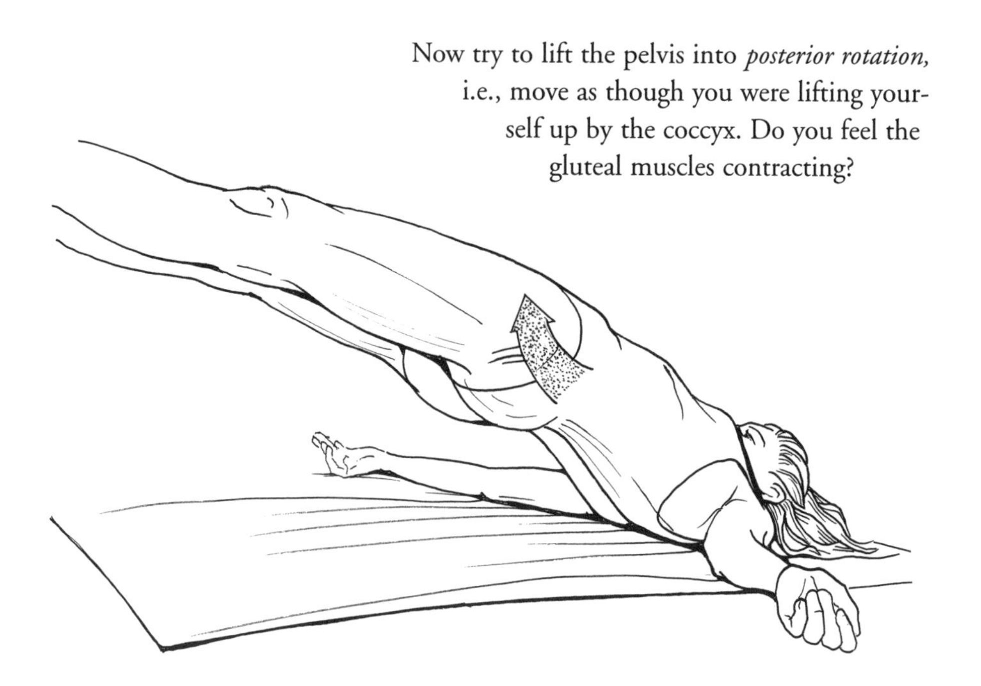

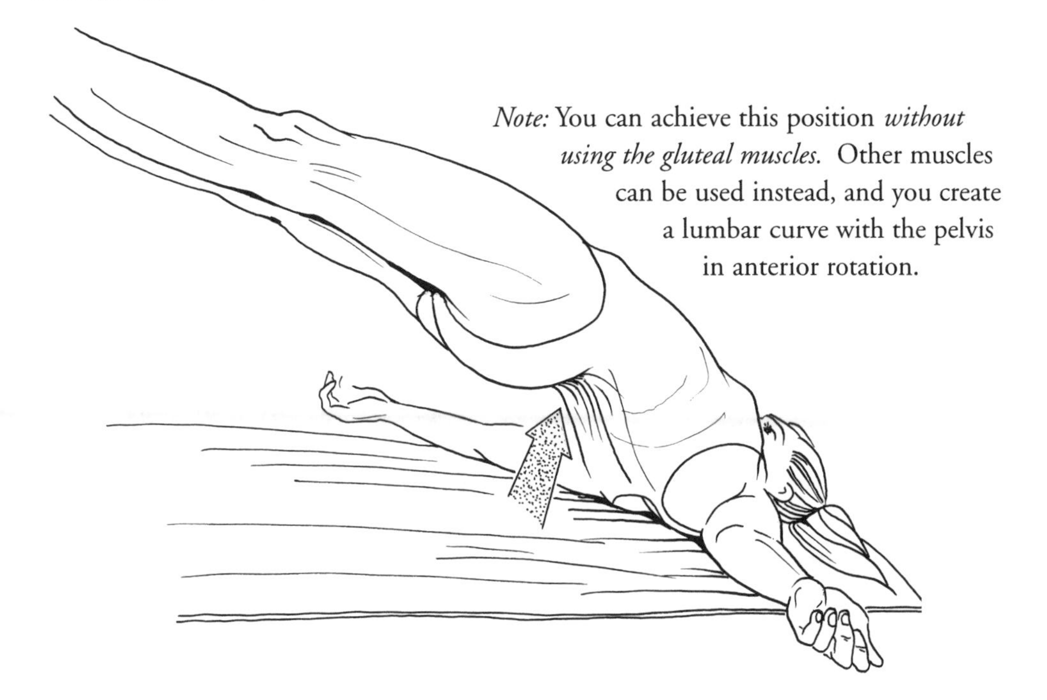

Note: You can achieve this position *without using the gluteal muscles.* Other muscles can be used instead, and you create a lumbar curve with the pelvis in anterior rotation.

2. Differentiating between the gluteal and pelvic floor muscles

The opening positions for this exercise and the previous one are identical. First, lift the body slowly by using the gluteal muscles, and then tuck in your tail, i.e., tilt (rotate) the pelvis backward. Remain a moment in this position and contract the pelvic floor muscles. It may help if you make short exhalations during this movement. Now relax the muscles completely and lower your back to the ground once more, slowly allowing yourself to be carried by the gluteal muscles.

3. Intensive version

Repeat the preceding exercise. When you have lifted up as far as you can, lift one foot up from the stool. The corresponding gluteal muscle is no longer in contraction, and the one on the other side has to work twice as hard. In this way, you can strengthen your gluteal muscles.

These exercises are particularly useful during pregnancy, especially if there is instability in the pelvic region. Remember that a change in the hormonal balance during pregnancy can sometimes make the joints overly mobile. The strengthened gluteal muscles will help stabilize the pelvic region. In addition, these exercises can also help during painful menstruation.

Exercises for the adductor muscles

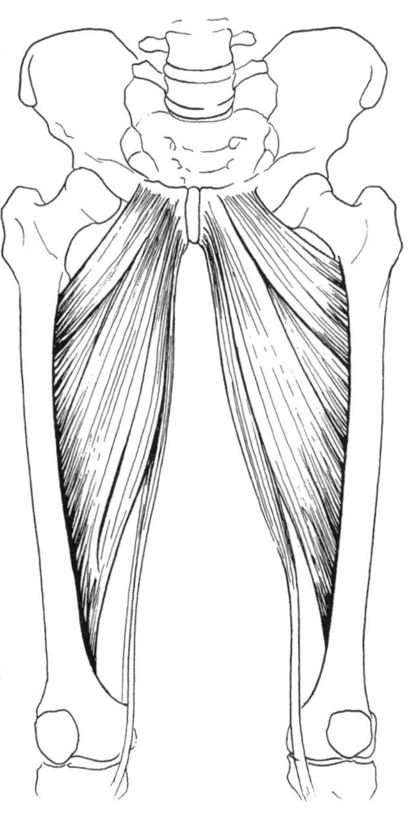

1. Locating the muscles

This exercise is from daily life:

Sit on a chair next to a table with one knee placed against the table leg. Now push your knee against the table leg as though you were pulling it toward the other knee. Be careful not to push your foot down to the ground, as that would bring other muscles into play.

Try to identify what produces the movement. You should be feeling the contraction of the muscles on the inside of your thigh. You can actually place your hand on them and feel the movement as they contract.

Now do the same exercise again, but each time, contract the muscles at a point higher and higher up along the thigh, and even try to relax the lower muscles. In this way, *you will activate the upper, deeper adductor muscles,* those closest to the pelvic floor.

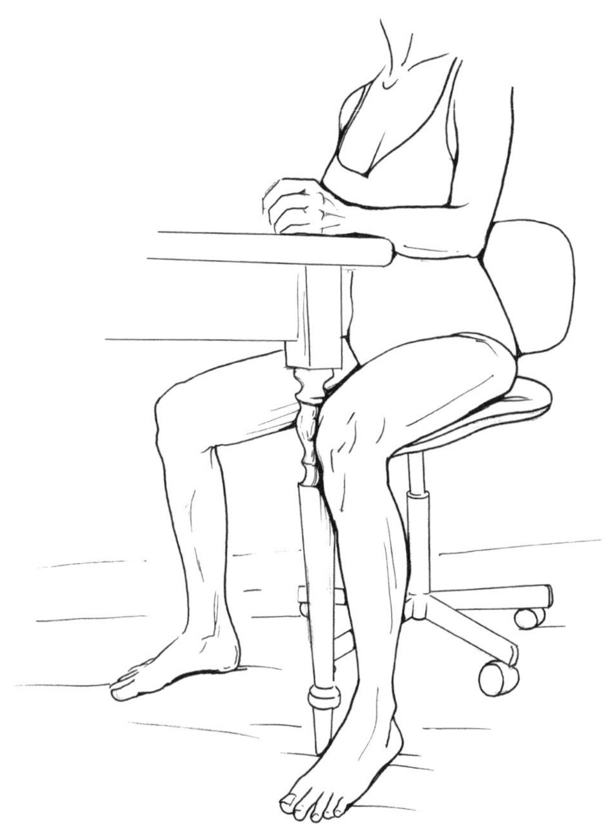

2. Distinguishing the perineum from the adductor muscles

Maintaining the same position, release the contracted muscles and now contract the perineum (see pp. 108-117). Do you feel how close the contractions are in this region? Only the ischiopubic ramus separates the two sets of muscles.

3. Stretching and strengthening the deep muscles of the internal femoral region

Repeat the first exercise on the previous page and hold the contraction for a couple seconds, then relax for twice as long. Now swing your chair around so that you are sitting with the thighs stretched apart. Stretch out as far as you can without going beyond your limit. Repeat the exercise. You will notice that after being contracted, the thigh will stretch out more easily. Thanks to this contract-relax exercise, you will have increased the mobility of your hip joint as well.

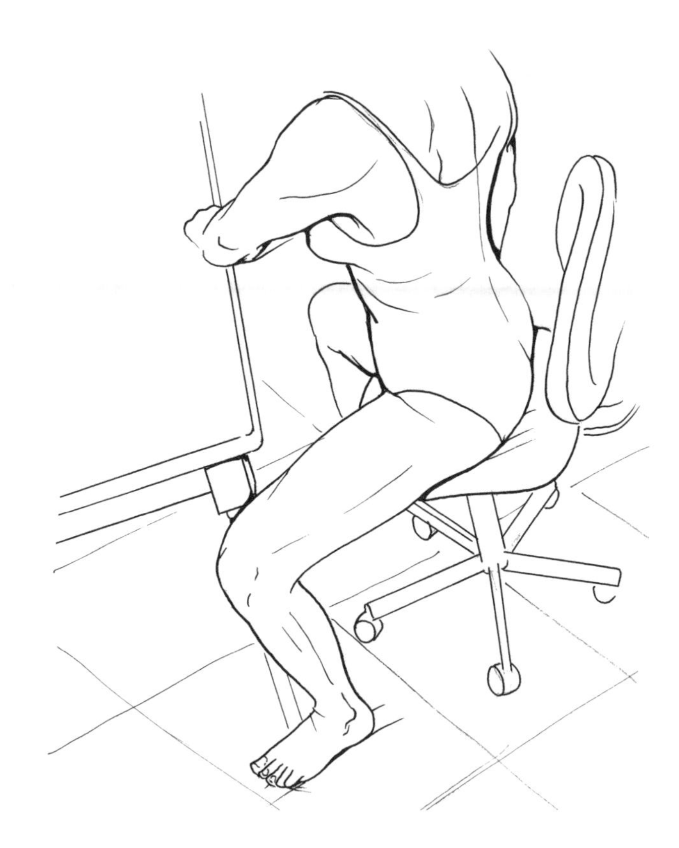

You can repeat this exercise as often as you like. You will be stretching and strengthening each of the deep adductor muscles at the same time.

4. Stretching out all the adductor muscles

To prepare yourself for the positions you will need on the day of delivery, try from time to time to find other positions that stretch out the inner thigh muscles, and at the same time keep the hip muscles flexible.

For example:

1. In a squatting position, open out the knees as wide as possible, then do a sideways stretch with one leg by straightening one knee and placing the heel on the ground out to the side.
2. Alternate from side to side, using your elbows to push your knees as far apart as you can.

The organs of the lesser pelvis

Exercises for the bladder and urethra

1. Feeling and recognition

Remember that the clearer you are about the sensations that you discern, and the mental image that you form, the better your movements will be. To start with, these exercises, which are to be practiced over a number of days, are intended to train your recognition of the different sensations involved.

Locating your urinary opening: This opening is situated between the labia minora, half a centimeter below the clitoris and above the vaginal opening. It often protrudes a bit.

Locating the ureter: The next time you urinate, try and locate the internal pathway followed by the urine. The sensation—a feeling of sliding—may well be felt as the urine passes through the muscular passage. Try to vary the force with which you urinate in order to create contrasting sensations (this is, however, not something to be practiced habitually, just from time to time).

Focus on the entire flow. Try to focus on this sensation during the entire time of urination. Especially be aware of the feeling when the flow starts, its strength, and the end of the flow.

Pay attention to when and where the urge to urinate arises. This will be found at the base of the bladder, at the origin of the urethra. You've probably become so accustomed to these moments, which can occur five or six times a day, that you no longer pay attention to them—you either urinate, or you wait and the sensation disappears. Now try and "program" yourself to catch the sensation and to recognize it from the moment it begins, i.e., the slight stinging feeling that occurs at a very precise location—the trigone—at the base of the bladder where the urethra originates, and within the urethra itself.

Similarly, as you urinate, recognize how the sensation gradually disappears as the bladder empties.

2. Forming a mental image of the bladder and urethra

Once you are able to recognize these different sensations, try, when you are not actually urinating, to establish the link with the rest of your anatomy.

You can begin by visualizing the passage of urine, starting from the external opening of the urethra in the perineum. Then go upward about five to six centimeters, backward and behind the pubic symphysis. When you are standing, the ureter is almost vertical as it rises obliquely toward the back.

You can also try to visualize the bladder as it changes its volume. The empty bladder is in the lowest anterior part of the abdomen, behind the pubic symphysis, and rises above the pubis when it is full.

Now try to visualize the bladder and urethra in other positions, e.g., when you are lying on your back, stomach, or side. What is their orientation? For example, when you are lying on your back, the urethra is oblique and points downward toward the ground. If you are on your stomach, it is oblique from bottom to top and rises toward the back.

If need be, help yourself by referring to the illustrations on pp. 46 and 48. Then turn the illustrations around to visualize their location as you assume different positions.

3. Active exercises for the urethra

When you have mastered the previous visualizations and exercises, you can proceed to the next step of active exercises. For these you can either lie down on your back, sit up, rotate the pelvis into anteversion, or (later on) take up the squatting position with your knees apart. These exercises are intended to be performed between urinations.

Try to contract the external sphincter of the urethra. To do this, squeeze the urethra as though you wished to flatten it out. Don't be surprised if, at the start, you contract the other two sphincters—the vagina and the anus—especially as the urethral sphincter is the smallest opening of the three, and the most difficult to differentiate. In addition, the urethral sphincter is situated just where the muscles form the urogenital hiatus, where muscular sensations are far weaker.

Don't worry if the other two sphincters contract at the same time. Use that as your baseline to gradually distinguish one set of sensations from the other.

Try to contract the urethra as though you were closing off a tube. Do this even if the feeling is only vague or confused with other muscular actions. Hold this for about five seconds.

Now relax completely for twice as long, breathing deeply. Repeat this exercise a number of times.

Now try different approaches. For example, squeeze only the urethra, contracting it:

- along its entire length (6-7cm)
- for longer periods, say six seconds, then release for twice as long
- as strongly as possible for a short space of time (only two seconds).

Eventually, you can try to contract the sphincter while the abdominal muscles are experiencing hyperpressure, e.g., while coughing, laughing, squatting, walking, or jumping (see p. 76).

Note: Always follow every contraction by a moment of complete relaxation that is twice as long as the contraction, and remember to breathe deeply. The reasons for this are:

- to increase your awareness of the different sensations by contrasting them, and
- to avoid hypertoning the sphincters.

4. Relaxing the urethra

This is something you can practice in order to relax the muscle you have just contracted, and also to amplify the action itself. Imagine that your urethra widens its diameter along its entire length, and hold that dilatation for a few seconds. (Don't be surprised if, at the same time, other parts of your body relax, even as far away as the mouth!) Just as with the contraction exercises, this relaxation exercise should be repeated many times in order that later you can do it at will.

Use this programmed relaxation of the urethra during urination and also for the exercises involving the bladder that we will look at later on. It is most important that the urethra open fully during urination, without any holding back.

5. Exercises for the bladder

Normal urination is one whose action you can control, either to start or to withhold. It should be easy and without discomfort or pain. It should be efficient, in other words, the bladder should empty completely without any deliberate assistance from abdominal pressure. Finally, it should not be too frequent—about five to eight times a day, and in some cases once a night.

There are many pathologies that can alter this normal function. In some cases, they will necessitate a medical diagnosis and treatment. However, every woman can cultivate an awareness of certain habits that usually go by unnoticed and that, although they are not serious, can upset normal function. Fortunately, there are simple enough remedies available.

Unfinished urination

For example, take a child who is obliged to interrupt a game to go urinate and who is in such a hurry to get back to the game that she doesn't take the time to completely empty her bladder. Adults can experience the same thing because of the pressure of professional activities or daily life. Another example is that of a pregnant woman who has a frequent need to urinate (see p. 51) and develops the habit of not completing the action because she thinks (sometimes quite unconsciously) that she will be back again before long anyway. In this way, a habit of never completely emptying the bladder develops, leaving a residue, which can become the source of urinary tract infections and a cause of frequent urination.

Take the time to observe your own habits, especially in the context of daily activities. If necessary, give yourself more time to finish urinating, however small the amount.

Forced urination

A person can develop the habit of pushing down on the bladder with the diaphragm and abdominal muscles (see p. 73), either because of stress, a desire to finish quickly, or an atonic bladder. Even if this action can help in those moments when you "haven't got time" to completely empty the bladder, don't let it become a habit. Normally, all that is needed to empty the bladder is the simple action of the bladder muscle itself.

Observe yourself: Do you let your bladder do the work when you urinate, or do you exert pressure from the abdomen? Is that pressure there from the start or the middle, or does it intervene only at the end?

In this situation as well, the exercise is simple and follows from your observations. If you always exert pressure, especially if you do it right from the start, try and form the following new habits:

- Wait, without pushing, and let urination occur passively, i.e., don't intervene. At the beginning, you may achieve this for only a moment, but then you will begin to notice that your bladder gradually takes charge of more and more of the action. Let the urethra relax (see p. 127) as the bladder contracts.
- Hold off pushing as long as possible once you start urinating, and then when you do push, try to do so as little as possible, no more than is absolutely necessary. You will begin to notice that the "final push" is no longer necessary; it is just a matter of your taking time.

Taking the time to urinate

The items below should encourage you to take into account your own lifestyle or circumstances, and to understand how they affect your urination. Here are some questions and suggestions:

- Is your toilet a pleasant place to visit, one that allows you to relax, think of your body, and take your time, or is it a place you want to get out of as fast as possible (like many institutional toilets)? Simple shifts in attitude could bring about remarkable changes.
- Do you personally recognize the importance of urinating and make space within your own life for this indispensable activity? This question evidently touches upon how each person thinks about and interprets this apparently simple act. This is a psychological question that is not within the bounds of this text, but it must be mentioned. This simple attention to you

bladder can make a big impact in the re-education of urgent urination. If these exercises don't make a difference, contact your physician.

"Pee-blocking"

We are talking here of consciously interrupting the flow of urine at a desired moment. No doubt you are already familiar with this well-known exercise. However, before you try to modify the strength of the muscles involved in urination, you should first be able to feel them clearly. If not, there is a risk of forcing the muscles in a haphazard manner.

A benefit of this exercise is being able to accurately feel the contraction within the urethra; if it is not felt in the urethra, the flow is not stopped! *But note:* If this exercise is misapplied, it can result in more disadvantages than advantages. There are a number of precautions to keep in mind:

- Do not do it at the onset of the urge to urinate, or while urinating.
- Do not do it more than once a day.
- Stop only once while urinating.
- Be sure to fully complete the urination.

Why take these precautions? *It is very important not to derail the urinary reflex.* After a while, if there is never enough urine left in the bladder, the urge to urinate could stop. This could bring about a situation of bladder instability (see p. 90) or urinary tract infections. Obviously, it is very important to maintain this important reflex. There is a similar danger if just a small volume of urine is left, which can likewise lead to urinary tract infections.

Follow the precautions listed above. There is no need to intensively train the bladder muscles!

So, how can you evaluate the strength of your urethral sphincters?

- A strong sphincter can completely stop the flow at the beginning of a strong urination.
- An average sphincter can stop the flow of a moderate urination relatively quickly.
- A feeble sphincter cannot stop urination, even with only a small amount of urine.

Exercises for the uterus and vagina

The uterus is not directly supported by muscles, but by the vagina, which is itself solidly attached to the levator ani muscle. The following exercises are therefore concerned with the vagina itself.

1. Awareness of the vaginal canal

Sensations within the vaginal region occur during different and very contrasting circumstances:

- during sexual relations
- during normal vaginal discharge
- during monthly periods
- while wearing a tampon
- during delivery.

In all of these circumstances (except possibly during a delivery), you can become aware of the feelings at the vaginal surface and visualize where the vagina is situated.

2. Forming a mental image of the vagina

Visualize the length of the vagina from the external orifice to its upper extent (approximately 10 centimeters) and its location between the urethra and the rectum (see Chapter 3). You should also think about its obliquity, i.e., if you are in an upright position, the vagina runs down from the back to the front of the pelvic cavity.

3. Forming a mental image of the uterus

Normally, the uterus lies forward over the bladder. When the bladder is empty, the body of the uterus lies in an oblique direction from back to front, and below to above (see p. 46). The vagina lies obliquely in the opposite direction, with the uterus being more horizontal. Just as you did for the bladder and the urethra, try locating the position and direction of the vagina and uterus in different positions:

- lying face down
- on your back
- on your side.

Make use of the drawings on p. 48 by turning them around on the page as you change positions.

4. Awareness and strengthening exercises for the pelvic floor muscles in the vaginal region

Sit down on any seat of chair height, with the pelvis tilted slightly forward (anteversion). Begin by repeating the exercises on pp. 112 and 113, which consist of raising the whole of the muscular structure of the pelvic floor containing the three main organs. Do you feel that you can make the contractions more specifically in the different parts of your pelvis:

- in front, to give more support to the urethra
- completely at the back, to support the anus and the rectum
- in the middle, to support and lift up the part between the two areas?

Try to contract the middle area even though you may feel that you cannot locate it precisely. Now imagine the vagina being placed not vertically, but obliquely, with the levator ani muscle pulling it even more obliquely toward the front.

5. Awareness and strengthening exercises for the vaginal muscles

The vagina is a tube that is normally flaccid and flattened by the pressure of adjacent organs, but it is a muscular structure with a muscular lining. The fact that it is muscular and has this double musculature is something most women don't realize. Here are some exercises for the vagina itself.

Longitudinal contractions

Because of the longitudinal fibers of the vaginal muscles, the vagina can shorten itself. Try to imagine the vagina segmented into three parts: bottom, middle, and top. Now imagine making a contraction that travels upward, as though you were folding the vagina. Begin the contraction close to the orifice, then include the whole of the lower segment. Hold this for a few seconds, then relax completely for a few seconds.

When you have clearly felt the contraction and can distinguish it from a pelvic floor contraction, try to move the middle segment. Hold that contraction for a few seconds, and again relax completely for a few seconds.

Now go further up again, as far as the top segment of the column, close to the cervix of the uterus. Keep in mind the image of an elastic tube shortening itself, which is quite different from the sensation you felt when the pelvic floor was used to lift the vagina. Remember to relax fully after each contraction. You may find that a contraction of the upper segment will cause the uterus to contract (see the exercise at the bottom of p. 115).

Contractions to the right and left of the vagina

The following exercise is important in helping you develop feeling in your vaginal area, by working from side to side.

Try to picture your vagina as having two halves, a left and a right. Contract the internal wall of the vagina along its entire length, but only on the right side. Try not to include the left side in the contraction.

Don't be surprised if at first this seems impossible or confusing, or if at this stage the contraction of the vagina causes other contractions elsewhere in the body, such as other muscles of the perineum, or in a suspension of your breathing. This is called *synkinesis,* and you will lose it little by little. Notice the sensations of the two sides at the same time: one side contracted and shortened, the other trying to stay long and relaxed. Gradually release the contraction.

Suggestion: To avoid confusion, you may prefer to wait until the following day before trying this exercise on the other side. Little by little, you will gradually be able to contract first one side, and then the other. Remember that the time for contraction should match the time for relaxation.

Sphincter-like contractions

The vagina can also narrow its width thanks to circular fibers that line its entire length. However, these fibers are found mainly in the lower section where they thicken into the vulval constrictors (see p. 53). Now try to close the orifice, blocking the entry to the vagina. Even if this sphincter is not as strong as those of the urethra and anus, it is nonetheless quite possible to strengthen it. Also, remember to relax completely after each contraction.

If you wear a tampon during your monthly periods, you probably make a similar small contraction to prevent the tampon from sliding out. The disadvantage of that kind of contraction is that sometimes you stay contracted too long and do not consciously take time to relax afterward.

Next, you can move upward to include the two lower segments of the vagina in the squeezing sphincter action.

Finally, use the contraction to reach the upper segment, as though you wished to close off the vagina at the level of the neck of the cervix. As always, hold the contraction for a few seconds, and then relax for the same amount of time.

6. Strengthening the uterine muscles

The contractions of the uterus during the latter part of pregnancy and during the actual delivery are often discussed. It is important to understand that contractions of the uterus need not necessarily be associated with or signify pain. Such contractions do occur under other circumstances as well, e.g., during orgasms or menstruation.

The uterus contracts during orgasms. Pregnant women can feel the contraction beneath the surface of the abdominal wall, just under the abdominal muscles.

During menstruation, the uterine epithelium detaches itself and is expelled from the uterus. Certain muscular fibers within the uterus contract more strongly than others, resulting in the sometimes painful sensation associated with menstruation. At the same time, the lower abdomen experiences *vasodilation,* giving the characteristic and sometimes painful sensation of heaviness.

In order to experience the events associated with menstruation more comfortably, and allow the body to function more efficiently, try the following simple exercises during menstruation:

- Lie down in a comfortable position on your back, or on your side if necessary, with your pelvis tilted slightly into retroversion with the help of a cushion. Do this for a few hours if possible (or for at least 15 minutes) during the day. This allows you to relax the muscles that would otherwise be working to maintain a standing posture.
- Cover yourself to keep warm, especially in the abdominal region. This will allow you

to relax the basic muscle tone since your body no longer needs to work so hard to keep itself warm.

All of this will help increase vasodilation and the expulsion of the menses. You may be surprised to find that as a result of these exercises, your blood loss will increase during menstruation (within limits), more so than if you participated in more strenuous activities. Active women who need to maintain their physical performance and tonicity for athletics may experience a reduction in their menstrual flow.

Exercises for the rectum and anus

Here, first try to become aware of the sensations in this region, then form a mental image of:

- the difference between the anus and the rectum
- the different types of movement of the rectum.

1. The reflex of defecation: locating the sensations

Early toilet training for some people is linked with the obligation to defecate "on command," and is therefore linked to pushing with the diaphragm (see blocked pushing on p. 73). This can upset the normal reflex action or the easy functioning of defecation.

The reflex action begins with a sensation of fullness in the rectum. This is such a normal and habitual feeling that it often passes quite unnoticed. The first thing to do is to be able to recognize the feeling associated with wanting to defecate, even if you are unable to do so right away.

Suggestion: Prepare yourself with a little advance programming the night before. Tell yourself that when the feeling does come, you will take note of it.

When the rectum is full, it feels stretched and heavy, a very distinct sensation. At the same time that you get this feeling, try to identify—using the feeling of heaviness—the position of the rectum, which is in the back third of the pelvic cavity (see p. 58).

2. Forming a mental image of the rectum

This discussion is not about the anus, which is much more superficial and lower down in the pelvic cavity. The rectum is situated five centimeters higher up, is approximately ten centimeters long, and four centimeters wide. It follows the curve of the sacrum and is concave toward the front.

As you have previously done for the urethra, take the time to identify the sensations associated with the rectum. You should not skip over this part of the exercise, which could take a number of days.

You will then become more clearly aware of the following eventualities:

- If an opportunity to defecate cannot be taken, then the sphincter contracts and the feeling of urgency is postponed.
- When you do have the opportunity to defecate, take a moment to identify another, more active sensation, that of the rectal sleeve contracting upon itself in order to begin evacuating the stool. This is the onset of the expulsion reflex.

3. Reeducating and strengthening the rectum

You should try to allow the rectum to do its job on its own, to expel the stool as the anus relaxes. In this case, you will not begin by pushing with the diaphragm. Try to delay pushing for a few moments and observe, as always, the sensations that appear.

The reason for postponing a diaphragmatic

push is to avoid using its strength to compress the stool downward in the rectum. When that occurs, the rectum becomes distended and will no longer be included in the expulsion of stool. It will contract much less since it is replaced by another muscle. In the long run, the rectum will become atonic.

In addition, compressing the stool may sometimes create too great a volume in the base of the rectum, provoking an extreme situation of compression and excessive stretching of the anal sphincter. This can cause pain and even hemorrhoids. It can also be the cause of excessive accumulation of stool in the rectum, as seen in some cases of constipation.

When the rectum is allowed to contract normally, it pushes out the stool through a narrowing along its entire length. This reduces the pressure on the anus since the overall volume is reduced. The process of defecation becomes easier when all that is required is for the striated sphincter to relax and not to become distended.

So take your time, and visualize the rectum shortening for a few moments (20-40 seconds) before pushing. By doing this very simple exercise, you will gradually notice that you have less need to push except in the final moment of expulsion. The rectal muscle itself will have regained tonicity and will be doing all the work.

4. Improving the tone of the entire length of the rectum

You can actively strengthen the rectal muscles by the following exercises, which, of course, are to be performed at moments not concerned with the action of defecation.

Longitudinal contractions

The muscular fibers of the rectum are capable of shortening along its entire length during contraction. Try to visualize the rectum along the sacrum and divide it into three segments—lower, middle, and upper—each of which is a little over an inch long. First, try to contract the lower fibers, those just above the anus, as if you were trying to withhold gas or stool. This will make the rectal passage move upward, as though squeezing in on itself. This is not the same sensation as the one you felt when you contracted the anal levator ani, which pulls up the rectum by pulling the anus toward the front (see p. 116). Hold the contraction for six to seven seconds, then relax completely. Do you feel how the weight stretches and pushes this region downward? Here as well, it is common to confuse the rectum with the neighboring areas. You will become more precise over time.

Next, try a contraction of the same type higher up, at the middle level. This part of the rectum is close to the sacrum, a little above the coccyx. Contract for a few seconds, then relax and breathe. To finish, contract the upper segment, around mid-sacrum. Again, relax and breathe.

Contraction of the circular fibers

By contracting the circular fibers you can narrow the space within the rectum, rather than drawing it upward. The circular fibers are a bit deeper than the others. Try to narrow the rectal tube throughout its length, dividing as before into three segments. Alternate each contraction with a few seconds of relaxation.

In these exercises, the most important part to strengthen is the first or lower segment. It is usually in this zone that the rectal passage becomes distended. Try the "drawing up" and "circular" exercises, concentrating on the front toward the vagina, and then on the back close to the coccyx. Always remember to relax between contractions.

These exercises are particularly helpful where there is distention of the rectum, lower bowel constipation (see pp. 91-92), onset of a rectocele (p. 92), or hemorrhoids (p. 93),[1] especially if they are associated with two other new habits:

- Trying to avoid pushing on a blocked breath, or at least waiting as long as possible before doing so.[2]
- Taking up a squatting position (or any similar position; see pp. 78-80) a few moments before sitting on the toilet. In this position, the rectum is slightly stretched from front to back as the distance between the coccyx and the pubis is increased. It is important to flex the thighs well and to lean the upper body well forward. This is where the hole-in-the-ground type of toilet has an advantage over modern toilets with seats. It is much better suited to the act of defecation.

When you repeatedly delay the passage of stool, the feeling that provokes the reflex disappears. This can be problematic if, during the day, you are obliged to repeatedly ignore the signal and end up using blocked-breath pushing to move the stool. If this happens every day, the reflex will become derailed and the rectal muscle will become inefficient.

In this way, a negative cycle is set up: The reflex is ignored and derailed, and defecation occurs on command, using the blocked-breath pushing method. If there is nothing you can do to change this situation on days when you're at work, it is even more important to use days when you're at home to practice the above exercises. Plan the night before so that you'll have enough time to pay attention to the sensations and actions of the organs involved.

5. Exercises for the anal sphincter

Start by either squatting or lying down on your back, with your knees drawn up.

Strong contractions

Try to contract the anal orifice as tightly as you can. The contraction should be felt at that level and not within the muscles of the pelvic floor (as you previously experienced when doing the vaginal exercises on pp. 112-117). Because the pelvic floor muscles span the pelvic cavity, contracting them will reflect the entire area. By contrast, contracting the anal sphincter alone, which is located in a very specific area, should feel like a small tube being tightened.

Longitudinal contractions

The sphincter muscle is about two centimeters in both thickness and length. Try to feel whether you can tighten it over its entire length. Hold for a few seconds, and then relax completely by breathing deeply. Repeat the exercise three or four times.

A more intensive exercise

Now repeat these exercises in daily situations associated with abdominal pressure (see p. 76). Remember to relax completely after each contraction.

This is an excellent practice if you are suffering from constipation or hemorrhoids since it helps increase the blood supply to the anal region, which is too often tense and distended by the pressure described in the last few pages. Not only will it help to strengthen the sphincter, it will also make it more resistant

1. Consult your physician should any of these occur.
2. Such pushing brings about very strong pressure on the anus, the posterior perineum, and the entire pelvic floor. If it is strong and becomes a habit, it can result in a prolapsed organ (see pp. 92-93).

to pressure, and more supple in those moments when it should expand.

6. Accepting the act of defecation

As with urination, notice how you experience this very basic action. Do you take the time and have the awareness necessary to enjoy the experience? Parental insistence during childhood to defecate on command and on being toilet trained, or referring to all that is dirty or shameful as "shit," can have a deep and sometimes disruptive influence on this simple act. Defecating (and urinating) is simply expelling something that cannot be assimilated by the body. It is not something that is bad in itself.

Decompressing the organs of the lesser pelvis

In standing (in other words, almost all day), the organs in the lower pelvis are subjected to constant compression, a situation accentuated sometimes by everyday activities (see pp. 76-77). In Chapter 3 we looked at the support and suspension systems that help the organs cope with compression. However, these systems can be damaged or the compression can increase or become prolonged, and thus painful. It is important to know how to alleviate this compression by finding positions of rest, or even of *active decompression.*

Decompressing by lying down on an inclined surface

If you lie down with the pelvis placed higher than the thorax, the pelvic organs will settle toward the top of the trunk. They will no longer be pressing on the perineum. Make sure that the whole body is on the inclined surface, e.g., by raising the foot of the bed. It is not enough just to put a pillow under the pelvis since that only produces a posterior rotation of the pelvis.

Decompressing by breathing

Lie down on your back on a comfortable surface with knees flexed and feet flat. Spread out your arms and place them so that the elbows are level with the shoulders.

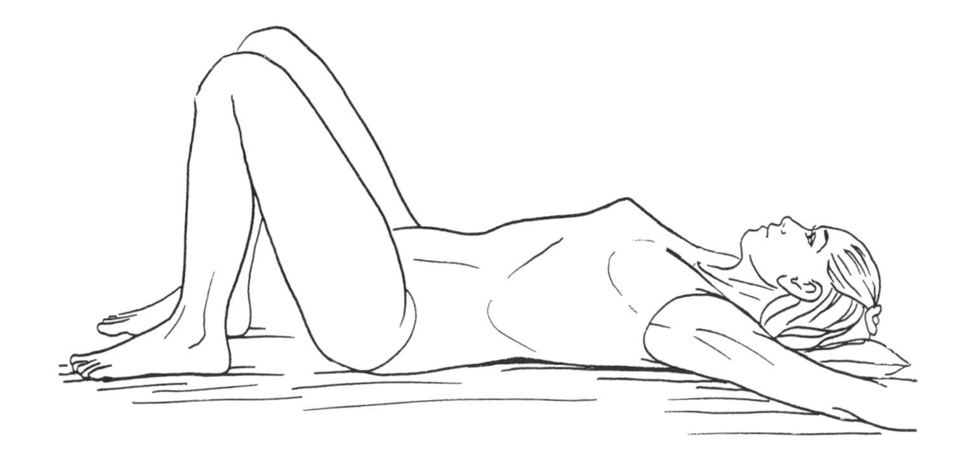

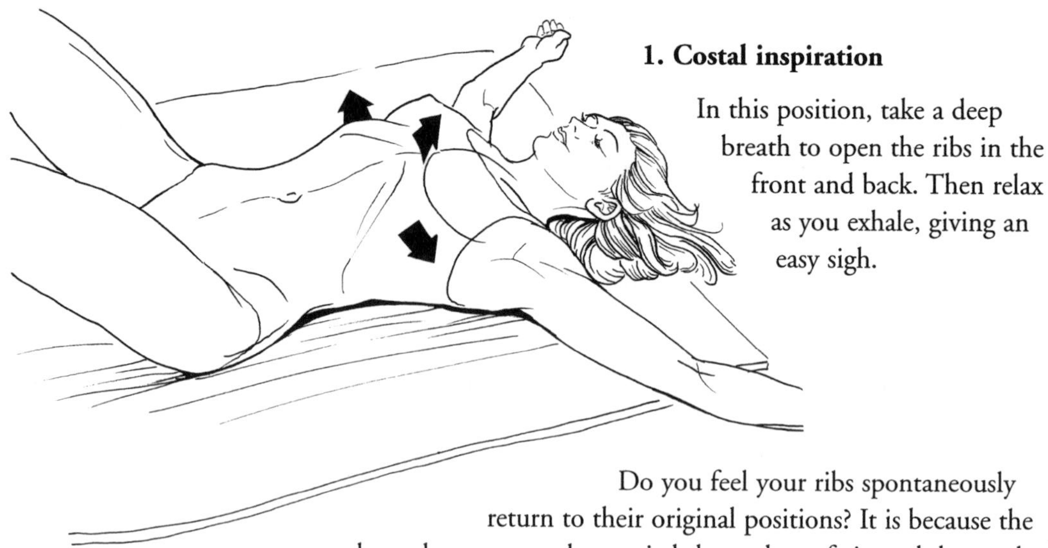

1. Costal inspiration

In this position, take a deep breath to open the ribs in the front and back. Then relax as you exhale, giving an easy sigh.

Do you feel your ribs spontaneously return to their original positions? It is because the lungs have retracted, emptied themselves of air, and drawn the ribs inward. Repeat this sequence a few times in order to feel the strength of the elastic return of the lungs, pulling the ribs back with them during exhalation.

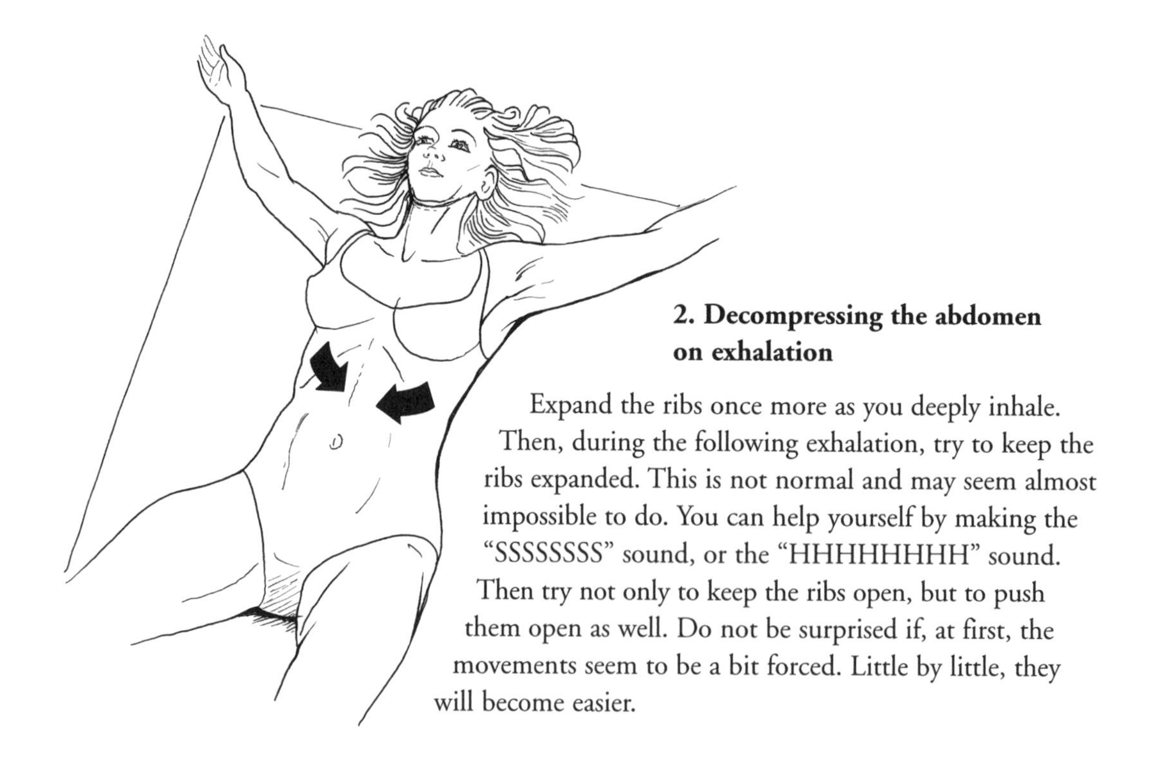

2. Decompressing the abdomen on exhalation

Expand the ribs once more as you deeply inhale. Then, during the following exhalation, try to keep the ribs expanded. This is not normal and may seem almost impossible to do. You can help yourself by making the "SSSSSSSS" sound, or the "HHHHHHHH" sound. Then try not only to keep the ribs open, but to push them open as well. Do not be surprised if, at first, the movements seem to be a bit forced. Little by little, they will become easier.

Do you feel as though the abdomen is being pulled toward the thorax? Because the lungs are no longer able to pull the ribs in with them, they now pull the abdominal mass itself upward. This creates a kind of *abdominal vacuum* that decompresses the lower organs.

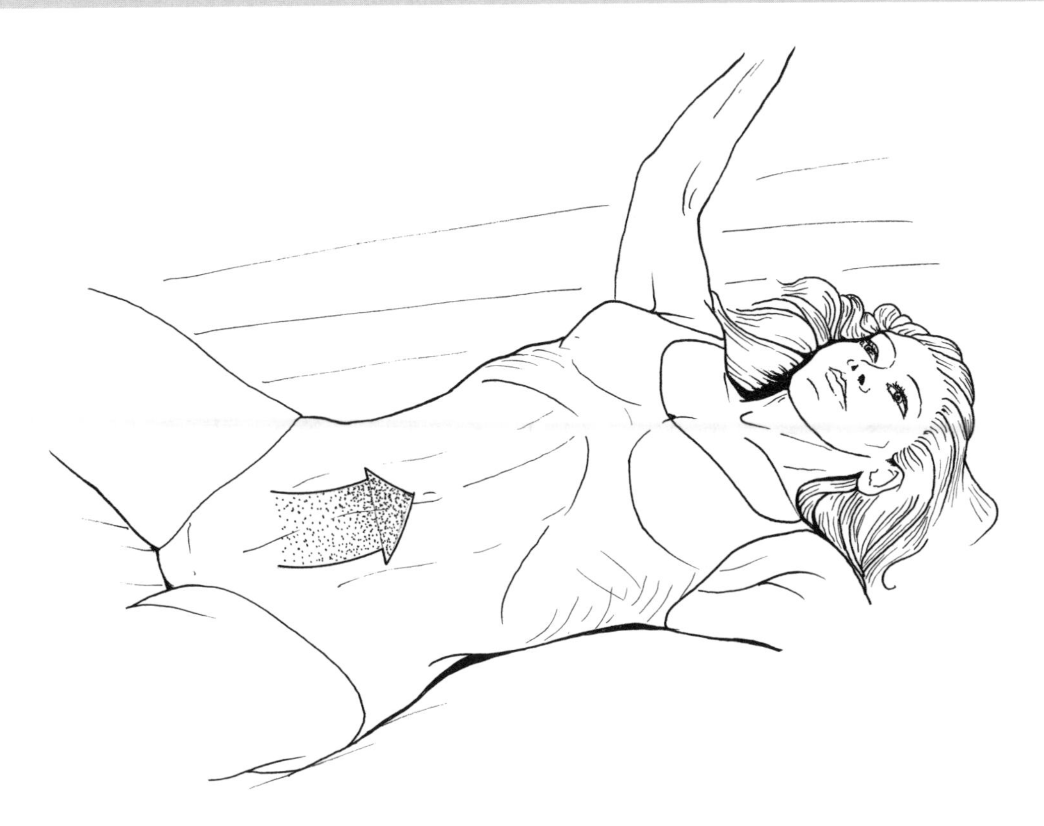

3. Aiming the zone of decompression

Now you can try to direct this zone of reduced pressure wherever you want in the abdomen, e.g., to the right or left, but more to the point, higher or lower. Imagine that your abdomen is divided into three levels:

1. an upper level, above the umbilicus
2. a middle level, just below the umbilicus, and
3. a lower level, that reaches as far down as the lesser pelvis.

Breathe again with the ribs expanded. Can you pull up the upper level of the abdomen, which is the most difficult to do? Can you feel and mobilize the entire region below the umbilicus? Can you mobilize the contents of the lesser pelvis? You need to do this very gently, pulling upward through the deep, internal center of the body.[1]

4. Suppressing neighboring effects (synkinesis)

You've probably noticed that other muscles come into play to pull up the pelvic organs. These are the abdominal muscles, the levator ani muscle, and the gluteal muscles. Try to locate and relax them wherever you can in order to concentrate on the traction of the pelvic organs by the lungs alone.

---

1. This location has a name in many different cultures, e.g., *dan tian* in China and *hara* in Japan.

5. Decompression centered on just one organ

Form a clear mental image of the organs in the lower pelvis (pp. 44-58). Now try to use the exercise to pull up either:

- the bladder and the urethra (without contracting the abdominal muscles)
- the uterus and the vagina (take care to relax the levator ani)
- the rectum and anus (keep the buttocks and the anal sphincter relaxed).

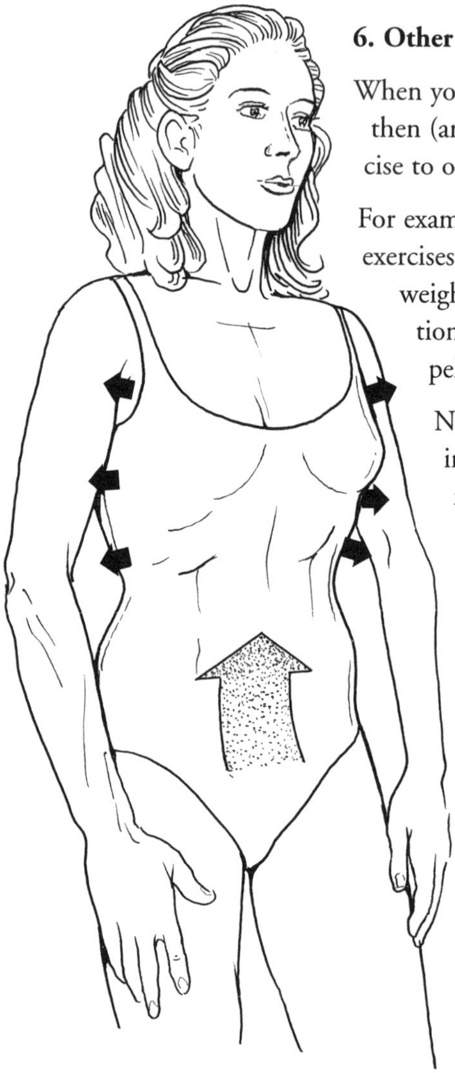

6. Other positions and situations

When you've become familiar with all of the previous stages, then (and only then) you can begin to transpose the exercise to other positions.

For example, what changes do you feel when you do these exercises standing up as opposed to sitting on a chair? The weight of the organs pulls them downward, and the position of the thighs can increase the involvement of the pelvic floor.

Now try a squatting position. Here the compression in the lesser pelvis is much greater and the exercise is more difficult to execute.

The best thing is to be able to do these exercises in ordinary, everyday situations.

They are useful for mobilizing the pelvic organs and for relieving the pressure that is placed on them. You can practice these exercises in a catch-as-catch-can manner during the day, no matter where you are, just to find the feeling; or you can practice them more intensively and repetitively during a planned exercise session. If your organs are particularly heavy or if are beginning to prolapse, it will be helpful to combine these exercises with mobilizations of the pelvic bones (see pp. 94-101).

Note: These exercises are especially recommended for the postpartum period. It is best to avoid them during pregnancy, as they could disturb the fetus.

CHAPTER NINE

Guidelines

How to protect the perineum before, during, and after delivery

The following pages review the contents of this book and discuss the precautions to be followed in different circumstances. The effects on the bony pelvic structure, the perineal musculature, and the internal organs of the lower pelvis will be examined, outlining the exercises that should or should not be done.

Note: These guidelines deal only with aspects directly concerning the perineum. There are, of course, many other related aspects to consider, but they are outside the scope of this work.

For the post-puberty period

This is the period from the end of puberty until a woman's first pregnancy, or if there is no pregnancy, right up to menopause.

Usually, until there is a pregnancy, the perineum is not really tested. In that case, you can read through this book simply as a guide to a region of the body about which you have, perhaps, relatively little knowledge. Of course, you will be able to practice all the exercises, except as advised on p. 94.

The situation is different if you have a lifestyle where your perineum is often subjected to heavy pressure, as described on p. 76. Three situations in particular bear mentioning because they are relatively frequent, and sometimes surprising:

- intensive sports
- an "hourglass" waist as a result of the development of the abdominal muscles (see p. 69)
- frequent coughing as a result of a respiratory pathology.

In such cases, your perineum needs a lot of attention, and perhaps even preventive care. A thorough understanding of the body and a sense of body awareness will be required to achieve the proper conditioning of the entire muscular structure and prevent the onset of the pathologies discussed on pp. 89-93, as well as prepare the perineum for pregnancy.

Use the practical exercise pages to exercise the perineal muscles (see pp. 108-117) and to develop a high degree of coordination between the perineal and abdominal musculature (see pp. 118-120).

For the duration of the pregnancy

During pregnancy, your body undergoes considerable changes, particularly with regard to the pelvis, abdomen, and breasts. It is most important to integrate each detailed exercise into a global awareness of your whole body by:

- forming a mental image of the significance of each area in relation to the overall body
- doing movements that involve the whole body, such as stretching and breathing exercises
- incorporating exercises into your daily routine.

THE PELVIC BONES

At the beginning of the pregnancy

During this period, the pelvis is sometimes unstable. If there is excessive movement between the three main pelvic bones (pp. 28-29), you could experience pain in the joints, for example:

- in the pubic symphysis
- in the sacroiliac joints (in the "small" of the back). This could have repercussions on the sciatic nerve, which lies right in front of the articulation. In this case, in order to *stabilize the pelvis during this period,* it may be useful to reinforce the muscles of the buttocks (see exercises on pp. 122 and 123). This can be done up to the eighth month.

In the middle and at the end of pregnancy

During these periods, you should perform the following exercises:

- those that increase the mobility of the pelvis, which will help the passage of the fetus through this area
- those that increase the mobilization of the pelvis in relation to neighboring structures, namely anterior/posterior rotation exercises and arching and stretching routines (see pp. 102 and 103)
- those that lead to a better understanding of the changes within the pelvis (see pp. 81-

83). Ideally, you should familiarize yourself with these exercises, identify those that suit you best while not neglecting the others, and experiment with different kinds of supports, e.g., cushions and stools

The day of delivery is too late to learn these exercises, and needless to say, *learning them before the delivery will allow you to determine the positions best suited for you* at that important moment. By preparing in advance, you will be ready with a small list of accessories to take with you that can add greatly to your comfort. For example, you may wish to take something to support your heels when you are in the squatting position (see p. 80). Maternity wards will not necessarily have thought of providing such supports for you.

THE PELVIC FLOOR MUSCLES

Because of hormonal changes that occur during this period, the connective tissue of the pelvic joints temporarily becomes more pliable. (This is true of all the connective tissue, including that of the pelvic floor).

To this is added the ever-increasing weight of the uterus, which is putting pressure on the lower pelvis. As a result of these changes, the perineal region may begin to feel heavy and distended. For this reason, it is even more important to repeat the exercises regularly (see pp. 108-117). Five to six minutes a day would be appropriate.

Conditioning of the pelvic floor presents a couple of advantages:

- It prevents muscular distention while promoting good tone.
- It prepares the musculature for adapting well to the compression and stretching associated with delivery.

To cultivate these results, respect the rule repeated throughout the exercise pages: Always follow muscle contractions with equal periods of relaxation.

THE DIAPHRAGM, ABDOMINAL, AND PELVIC FLOOR MUSCLES

Practice coordinating the muscles you will use at the bearing-down phase of the delivery, experimenting with the different ways of pushing described on pp. 73-74, but without overdoing it. It is really important to know how to do this before the delivery, not just theoretically, but through *actual repetitions* that will eventually give you an instinctive feeling for what to do when the moment arrives.

From the beginning of the pregnancy, practice distinguishing how pressure from the diaphragm can be directed to one or another of the orifices of the lower pelvis. Every so often, when you go to the toilet, you can practice pushing the flow of urine, what is called a *controlled push.* Never use force. Instead, try to feel how you can *direct the pressure* directly toward the bladder and not toward the anus. Conversely, when defecating, try to create a gentle but very precise pressure toward the rectum and anus without pressing on the bladder. Be careful not to overdo these exercises. Rather, *practice them just enough to be able to use them.* Under normal circumstances, urination and defecation are performed without pressure from the diaphragm.

Never push toward the uterus and vagina. Instead, simply imagine a line of pressure directed toward that area, and on the day of delivery, you can direct the pressure—maybe just mentally—toward that area. The direction of the push required here is quite different from the direction used when pushing while defecating. If the latter direction were used here, the fetus would be pushed heavily against the posterior perineum and the central tendon of the perineum (see p. 42). By practicing the simple exercises outlined here, you may be able to avoid distending the perineum or requiring an episiotomy (see p. 42).

Considering an epidural?

Pay special attention to the sensations you experience while doing the above exercises. You can try naming them so that you can lead the movements and feel them while you're doing them. You may wonder why you need to do this. It is because the epidural will not only alleviate the sensation of pain, it will also change or diminish other sensations, such as contracting and/or stretching. During the bearing-down phase, this will not necessarily make it easier for you to participate in the movements. However, if you prepare yourself in advance by focusing on the relationship between the sensations and their resulting effects, you will be able to remember them, even in a diminished state, and use them to participate in the delivery.

THE INTERNAL ORGANS

Bladder

From the fourth month on, the uterus begins to compress down on the bladder, resulting in more frequent urination. When this occurs, follow the simple rule: *Empty the bladder totally, even if there is only a small amount, without pushing, in order to preserve the urination reflex mechanism* (see p. 50).

Practice the exercises (see pp. 126-129) for heightening your awareness and increasing the tone of the urethra and bladder before delivery. This will help, however little, to keep the muscular tissue in good condition. The urethra will be greatly stretched during the fetal descent (see p. 51), and these exercises will prepare it to withstand the pressure.

Uterus

As the baby grows, the uterus gets larger and larger. During pregnancy, especially in the final weeks, your body positions can influence fetal position. This could be vital for the actual moment of giving birth, and for your perineum (see pp. 82-83).

Why is that? If you choose mainly sitting or lying down positions, like resting on a seat or reading or knitting on a chaise lounge, the fetus, even in the head-down position, will tend to settle into a similar position, with its back sagging toward the back of your abdomen. This puts the face of the fetus forward, which could prolong the engagement of the head in the birth canal. Even though this "occiput posterior" position is a vertex presentation (see p. 87), it is not optimal because:

- the baby's face presents a much larger surface than the occiput, and
- a much larger rotation is needed to bring the occiput to the front.

It is much better for the fetus to present with the head facing the sacrum (occiput anterior). In this way, the smallest diameter of the baby's head engages the vulva, which makes the delivery easier for the baby and carries less risk of damaging the mother's perineum. In fact, certain positions, such as *forward-leaning positions,* can help the fetus achieve the desired presentation. The fetus will then tend to fall forward as though in a hammock, with its back facing the mother's abdomen and its head facing the sacrum.

Rectum

The small and large intestines are progressively pushed toward the back and sides of the abdomen by the ever-increasing size of the fetus. The mother's digestive process often slows down as a result, sometimes leading to constipation. This shows how important it is to practice regularly all the exercises that increase the tonicity of the anus and rectum (see pp. 132-135).

For the delivery

Read this section before the delivery, at least during the last few weeks of pregnancy. The day of delivery is too late!

RELAXING THE PERINEUM AND MAKING IT MORE SUPPLE

The term *expulsion* describes the last phase of delivery (see the description of the birthing process on p. 85). Even if the delivery takes a short amount of time, it nevertheless carries a risk of damaging the perineum. However, with some simple precautions and actions, you can prepare the perineum for this event.

By massaging the pelvic area

The perineum is still not totally stretched in the hours preceding the delivery, and you can use massage to render it more supple. Working along the external skin surface with two or three fingers of the hand, you can massage in any direction or in the direction of the muscle fibers that make up the central tendon of the perineum (see p. 36). Also think about massaging along the interior ischiopubic rami, the external sides of the labia majora, and the outside of the vulva and anus.

By bathing

This is good thing to do before the expulsion phase. A warm bath (not hot) or a hip bath for a quarter to half an hour generally increases the pliancy of the tissues and relaxes the muscles, particularly those of the perineum.

By using a warm compress

Use a folded towel, soaked in warm to hot water and wrung out, or a warm, dry towel applied to the perineum during the time just preceding the expulsion. The warmth and humidity will have a similar, if more subtle, effect as that of a bath.

Note: For practical and hygienic reasons, these techniques may be considered controversial in the maternity ward to which you are admitted. It is indispensable to discuss your wishes well in advance of your delivery date with your midwife or obstetrical team, and to anticipate any eventual practical arrangement that may arise during the delivery.

By adopting the bearing-down method to aid the expulsion

As we have seen on pp. 71-74, expulsion can be accompanied either by blocked pressure or by an exhalation that leaves the uterus to work alone.

Certainly, while each of these two variations has its advantages and disadvantages, it is important to remember that pushing on exhalation is less traumatic to the perineum. For it to really work, you must use the *expulsive reflex* (see page 71). And if one pushes too quickly, this reflex will not come into play.

Where to push when you bear down

Many women have a mental image of the events that occur in the middle of the perineum, and this notion is reinforced when they hear others say, "Push down as though you are going to the toilet."

This is exactly where a better knowledge of anatomy can really help you protect your own body. Take time to review the pages on the pelvis showing the shape of the three openings or orifices (pp. 17-24), the pelvic cavity (p. 25), and the perineum and superficial muscles (pp. 33 and 37). As you examine those illustrations, you will realize that the *fetus follows a curved path.* The exit is not in the center of the perineum, but in the anterior perineum. To be even more precise, the vaginal orifice is not next to the pubic symphysis, but is set back a little within the anterior perineum.

This small detail can help you follow the baby's exit *without pushing too much:*

- toward the back, which could stretch the central tendon, or
- toward the front, thereby avoiding putting pressure on or distending the urethra.

To summarize, do *not* push:

- straight down
- as though you were going to the toilet
- toward the pubis.

But you *should* push toward the vaginal opening. Does this seem impossibly precise? It is for this very reason that we presented exercises to help you feel exactly where to direct your efforts!

When to stop pushing

During the delivery, you may be asked to stop pushing. This is because it is possible, without endangering the baby, to slow down the expulsion when there is a risk of over-stretching the perineum by applying too much pressure. In this situation, it is very important, even if you feel a strong desire to push, to suspend your efforts as much as you can for the sake of your perineum.

For the postpartum period

Postpartum refers to the period following delivery, and can be divided into two stages:

- The first eight to twelve days after delivery when all the structures have been very heavily stretched and are in the process of healing. During this period, you must take great care not to do too much.
- The weeks following this first stage when you will be able to gradually increase your exercise and tone your perineum.

Ask your maternity service for a routine check of your perineum as well as recommendations for toning, if necessary.

PELVIC BONES

The delivery can cause unusual stretching movements between the pelvic bones. They can then remain in various positions that could adversely affect the normal balance of this region. It is advisable to have the balance restored by osteopathic manipulation. In addition, wait for at least six weeks before practicing the exercises to mobilize the pelvis described in Chapter 8.

PELVIC FLOOR MUSCLES

Depending on the delivery, the muscles of the perineum can become stretched, distended, or even torn. For this reason, it is important that any contractions should be made progressively and with *absolutely no abdominal pressure.*

You can repeat the exercises presented on pp. 109-111 and the second exercise on p. 112, but do them gently, just enough to activate contraction of these muscles. Repeat them a number of times each day, for instance, during breast-feeding or when giving the bottle. Choose easy, lying-down positions rather than the squatting positions you would use for more intensive exercising.

ABDOMINAL MUSCLES

We have seen (p. 69) that abdominal exercises can bring about too much pressure on the perineum. The abdominal organs gradually fall back into place postpartum just as the muscles regain their tonicity. However, the overall balance is fragile. Many women are in a hurry to get their stomachs "flat" again, but it is inadvisable to practice abdominal strengthening exercises until a good six weeks after delivery. Then you may begin practicing abdominal strengthening exercises, but take care to follow the process suggested in the second and third exercises on p. 119. In other words, always begin abdominal strengthening by contracting the pelvic floor, and keep it contracted during the entire period you exercise the abdominal muscles. Postpartum, this type of strengthening and toning regimen can usually be taken care of in physical therapy. To start on your own, *avoid all situations that could create too much abdominal pressure,* in particular, any kind of lifting or carrying. Even though it may be necessary to carry the baby, stroller, or big bags of diapers, avoid it as much as possible (see p. 76).

You should *plan* the postpartum period well in advance of delivery and *organize* your daily routine in detail so that you will be able to avoid lifting and carrying for at least two months. The most useful exercises during this period are those for decompression of the internal organs through breathing (see pp. 135-138). You should repeat them a few times each day.

THE PELVIC ORGANS

Bladder and urethra

The bladder, and even more so the urethra, have probably been compressed and distended by the delivery, which could lead to a number of problems. Just after delivery, the sensations associated with the urge to urinate could be absent. When this happens, the bladder fills up and takes up too much room in the upper part of the pelvic cavity. This could hinder the uterus from returning to its natural position. Your physician should check for this condition.

A more long-term problem is that of not being able to hold back the flow of urine during the first couple months after delivery. The bladder may have descended: The pressure balance between the bladder and the uterus may have become inverted, leaving the bladder in a restricted position normally intended for the uterus. This can result in postpartum incontinence. This condition is usually transitory and disappears as all the pelvic structures gradually return to their places, as long as you avoid excessive pressure on the perineum during the first two months.

Uterus

This organ returns to its initial volume in a few hours. However, the suspensory ligaments, i.e., the round and uterosacral ligaments (pp. 56-57), have been stretched so the uterus may be badly pulled back or even retroverted. To encourage proper repositioning, it is a good idea to spend a bit of time lying down on your belly at the beginning of the postpartum phase, as the weight of the uterus will make it fall forward. Later on you can exercise on all fours, which will have the same effect (pp.102-103). You can also practice your pelvic floor muscle contractions in these positions. Remember to follow the following precautions:

- Do not lie face down on too soft a bed as this will induce too much lumbar curvature.
- Do not stay too long in this position if you feel any strain in the still-stretched abdominal muscles.

Rectum

The rectum may also have been distended during the delivery. Try as best you can to avoid becoming constipated at this time, and especially avoid pushing with the diaphragm when you defecate, which could lead to prolapse of one of the pelvic organs.

EPISIOTOMY OR TEAR

If you had an episiotomy or a tear, however small, pay attention to the following:

- Protect the wound from infection. When

urinating, tilt the pelvis forward, with the ischia pulled back to prevent the urine from running over the vaginal region.
- When defecating, remember to wipe the anus from *front to back* (not the reverse), to avoid stool coming into contact with the vagina.
- Try spraying the perineum with an atomizer filled with mineral water after each visit to the toilet.
- Wait a while before beginning pelvic floor exercises. The scar from an episiotomy requires special care, and you should wait until it is well-healed before beginning pelvic floor exercises again.

For the menopausal and postmenopausal periods

Around age fifty women enter menopause, a time when hormonal changes once again modify the state of the perineum. At this time, the muscles lose strength and elasticity, and are easily over-stretched. Many women complain of a feeling of heaviness in their abdominal region, around the vulva, and of a feeling similar to the contractions that preceded their monthly periods. These symptoms increase whenever there is excessive pressure on the perineum (see p. 76), such as when tired, after standing for long periods, or after prolonged physical activity.

Problems cited in the chapter on pathologies of the perineal region, such as urinary incontinence and prolapsed organs (see pp. 89-93), can begin to manifest during menopause. These are often the result of lesions produced during childbirth that were not noticed while the muscular tissue was still strong and elastic. The loss of the perineal muscles' tone and elasticity as a result of aging now reveals the problem. Understandably, if you suffered from urinary incontinence after childbirth, you run the risk of similar problems at menopause.

Certain things can be done to improve your general health during this period:

- Start preparing from about the age of forty-five by practicing the exercises in this book for developing awareness and tone. Use them with the aim of learning about this particular region of the body, becoming aware of your feelings, and recognizing the signs of fatigue or weakness. Also use them to maintain the strength and elasticity of your muscles.
- Try to avoid all situations that could provoke perineal prolapse, especially diaphragmatic pushing during defecation and urination. Most of all, try to avoid becoming constipated; seek medical treatment if necessary.
- During or even after menopause, increase the number of times you practice the prescribed exercises, especially those that build up the muscles (see pp. 108-117). Try to do the exercises during two ten-minute sessions twice a week, more if the state of your perineum requires it.
- Finally, try to incorporate the exercises into your daily life.

At this stage of your life, it is essential to learn to follow each contraction with a similar period of relaxation, and to breathe deeply and fully during all the exercises. Tissue quality is much improved by good oxygenation.

Index

In this index the use of the letter *f* after a page number indicates a figure in the text.

A

B

C

E

F

G

H

I

J

K

L

R

S

T

U

V

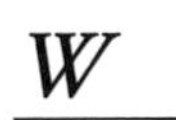